# Pocket Guide to
# LGBTQ Mental Health

## Understanding the Spectrum of
## Gender and Sexuality

# Pocket Guide to LGBTQ Mental Health

## Understanding the Spectrum of Gender and Sexuality

Edited by

**Petros Levounis, M.D., M.A.**

**Eric Yarbrough, M.D.**

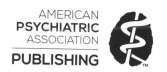

AMERICAN
**PSYCHIATRIC**
ASSOCIATION
**PUBLISHING**

If you wish to buy 50 or more copies of the same title, please go to www.appi.org/specialdiscounts for more information.

Copyright © 2020 American Psychiatric Association Publishing

ALL RIGHTS RESERVED

First Edition

Manufactured in the United States of America on acid-free paper

24   23   22   21   20      5   4   3   2   1

American Psychiatric Association Publishing

800 Maine Avenue SW

Suite 900

Washington, DC 20024-2812

www.appi.org

**Library of Congress Cataloging-in-Publication Data**

Names: Levounis, Petros, editor. | Yarbrough, Eric, 1979– editor. | American Psychiatric Association, issuing body.

Title: Pocket guide to LGBTQ mental health : understanding the spectrum of gender and sexuality / edited by Petros Levounis, Eric Yarbrough.

Description: First edition. | Washington, D.C. : American Psychiatric Association Publishing, [2020] | Includes bibliographical references and index.

Identifiers: LCCN 2020007953 (print) | LCCN 2020007954 (ebook) | ISBN 9781615372751 (paperback ; alk. paper) | ISBN 9781615373109 (ebook)

Subjects: MESH: Sexual and Gender Minorities—psychology | Sexual Behavior | Sexuality | Gender Identity | Counseling—methods | Handbook

Classification: LCC RC451.4.G39 (print) | LCC RC451.4.G39 (ebook) | NLM WM 34 | DDC 616.890086/6—dc23

LC record available at https://lccn.loc.gov/2020007953

LC ebook record available at https://lccn.loc.gov/2020007954

**British Library Cataloguing in Publication Data**

A CIP record is available from the British Library.

# Contents

# Contributors

**Murat Altinay, M.D.**
Assistant Professor of Medicine and Staff Psychiatrist, Cleveland Clinic Foundation, Cleveland, Ohio

**Adrian Jacques H. Ambrose, M.D., M.P.H., FAPA**
Child and Adolescent Psychiatrist, Massachusetts General Hospital, Harvard Medical School, Boston, Massachusetts

**Mary E. Barber, M.D.**
Clinical Assistant Professor, Columbia College of Physicians and Surgeons, New York, New York

**E.K. Breitkopf, M.A.**
Doctoral candidate, The New School for Social Research, New York, New York

**Serena M. Chang, M.D.**
Associate Director of Psychiatry, Callen-Lorde Community Health Center; Clinical Assistant Professor, Department of Psychiatry and Department of Child and Adolescent Psychiatry, New York University, New York, New York

**Victoria Formosa, L.C.S.W.**
Psychotherapist, Behavioral Health Department, Callen Lorde Community Health Center, New York, New York

**Selale Gunal**
Senior, Hunter College High School; American Museum of Natural History Brown Scholar, New York, New York

**Petros Levounis, M.D., M.A.**
Professor and Chair, Department of Psychiatry, Rutgers New Jersey Medical School; Chief of Service, University Hospital, Newark, New Jersey

**Sam Marcus, M.A.**
Doctoral candidate, The New School for Social Research, New York, New York

**Mark Joseph Messih, M.D., M.Sc.**
Child and Adolescent Psychiatry Fellow, University of Rochester Medical Center, Rochester, New York

**Ahmad A. Mohammad, M.D., M.S.**
Resident Physician, Maimonides Medical Center, New York, New York

**Sarah Noble, D.O.**
Medical Director, Outpatient Behavioral Health Einstein Medical Center, Philadelphia, Pennsylvania

**Angeliki Pesiridou, M.D.**
Director of Psychiatry, Callen-Lorde Community Health Center, New York, New York

**Daena L. Petersen, M.D., M.P.H., M.A.**
Psychiatric Services Director of HIV Psychiatry and Gender and Sexuality, Berkeley County Mental Health Center, South Carolina Department of Mental Health; Staff Psychiatrist, Berkeley Community Mental Health Center, Moncks Corner, South Carolina

**Eric Yarbrough, M.D.**
Private practice, New York, New York

**Nix Zelin, M.D.**
Founding member and vice president of the Northeast Student Queer Alliance, Moraga, California

## Disclosures

*The following contributors have indicated that they have no financial interests or other affiliations that represent or could appear to represent a competing interest with the contributions to this book:*

Adrian Jacques H. Ambrose, M.D.; E.K. Breitkopf, M.A.; Serena M. Chang, M.D.; Victoria Formosa, L.M.S.W.; Petros Levounis, M.D., M.A.; Sam Marcus, M.A.; Mark Joseph Messih, M.D., M.Sc.; Eric Yarbrough, M.D.

# Preface

*LGBTQ²IAPA*

What an acronym!

What are all these letters doing up there? What do they even mean? Are human beings really all that diverse? Well, yes. And probably much more than what this alphabet soup implies and what we have included in the little volume that you are now holding in your hands.

The purpose of this book is to help clinicians (as well as patients, parents, teachers, students, administrators, and anyone else who is interested in how humans operate) master the fundamentals of sexual orientation and gender identity. Building on our previous American Psychiatric Association Publishing books (Petros was the lead editor of *The LGBT Casebook*, with Jack Drescher and Mary Barber, back in 2012, and Eric wrote the *Transgender Mental Health* textbook in 2018), we have put together a pocket guide to the wonderful world of gender and human sexuality.

For this new edition, we have asked experts in the field of LGBTQ mental health to reflect on both the scientific literature and their own clinical experience in order to end up with a volume that aims to be informative, practical, and easy to read. The book is organized, very simply, in 10 chapters: lesbians, gay men, bisexuals, transgender people, queers, questioning people, intersex people, asexuals, pansexuals, and allied heterosexuals. Some chapters overlap because it is possible for one individual to identify with several of these identities. Each chapter begins with the psychological and cultural context of that particular facet of human sexuality, which includes history and definitions, as well as the twenty-first-century reality of the people who identify with the title of the chapter. We then address questions that well-meaning people may ask: What would patients, their friends, their parents, their physicians like to know about being X, Y, or Z? Finally, we discuss some common themes that may emerge in counseling and psychotherapy with LGBTQ²IAPA people.

And yes, you guessed it, we'll often abbreviate this terrific—but admittedly messy—acronym.

Society's understanding of gender and sexual orientation has changed dramatically in the late twentieth and early twenty-first centuries. When the gay civil rights movement symbolically started with the Stonewall Riots in New York City in 1969, LGBTQ people had been living in the closet since ancient times. Since then, a rainbow of gender and sexual identities has blossomed, giving each person the potential to express and identify themselves as they see fit.

Gender, previously thought to be strictly segregated into male and female, is now seen as a spectrum of many and sometimes fluid possibilities. The question is no longer whether someone is male or female but what masculine and feminine traits each of us possesses. We have added terms such as genderqueer, genderfluid, gender nonbinary, intersex, and transgender to our understanding of how people live, love, work, and play.

Sexual orientation has also evolved to encapsulate the diversity of sexual identity, sexual behavior, and sexual attraction. Most people used to identify as straight or gay, but many are now adopting the identities of bisexual, pansexual, asexual, queer, and questioning. Also, how someone identifies does not necessarily imply how they behave sexually or what their sexual attractions may be. For example, men who live on the "down low" identify as straight and sleep with both men and women, and their sexual attraction falls closer to the homosexual than the heterosexual end of the Kinsey scale.

Although the range of individual expression has grown over the past decade, equality and basic civil rights are far from being guaranteed for those who are gender and sexually diverse. Society continues to separate people into categories, placing higher value and protections on those who fit the "traditional" notion of what it means to be human. We hope that this book will demystify some of the complexities of gender and sexuality, making our world a more accepting and inclusive place.

We would like to thank American Psychiatric Association Publishing for the opportunity to present this pocket guide to you and for providing space for topics that are often underrepresented. This book would not be possible without the exceptional contributions, dedication, and passion of our coauthors, who spend their daily work advocating and serving those who are most in need. We are also indebted to our patients, our colleagues, our teachers, and our students, who keep us both exhilarated and on our toes in the office, on the wards, and in the classroom. Finally, we would like to give a shout out to our families of origin and families of community: We love you, and we forgive you if you don't know the 10 letters in the acronym at the heart of our book.

*Petros Levounis, M.D., M.A.*
*Eric Yarbrough, M.D.*
Newark, New Jersey, and New York City
March 2020

orientations have high rates of exposure to workplace sexual harassment, as we have seen with the "Time's Up" and "Me Too" movements. Most states and institutions continue to discriminate against gay people, with some even allowing queer people to be fired from their jobs simply because of their identity. The civil rights progress made may seem fragile at times, and it remains easily threatened by certain political parties and leaders. Clinicians who want to provide sensitive care need to be aware of the current political climate and news, both local and national, that may affect the rights and safety of their LGBTQ+ patients.

The L in LGBTQ[2]IAPA stands for lesbian, an identity label used by some women who are attracted to women. With so many expressions of sexuality present around the world, different people choose to identify themselves in different ways, and lesbian is a term that has been often associated with western culture. In both this chapter and the following chapter about gay men, a variety of terminology will be presented for two main sexual identities that have evolved over time.

The origin of the word lesbian comes from the island of Lesbos and is associated with the Greek poet Sappho (c. 610–570 B.C.E.). It was originally adopted by women who love women and has been used over the past century in various ways. Recently, however, to a majority of queer women, the word lesbian sounds old-fashioned or unnecessarily separate from gay men, or it just doesn't fit for them. Many women are now choosing gay or queer as an identity label, whereas others embrace more diverse terms. The history of the LGBTQ+ community left many members feeling invisible, particularly queer people of color. Lesbians of color may choose such terms as BlaQ, BlaQueer, and stud, which they believe more fully describes them, their sexual orientation, race, ethnicity, and gender—an intersection of their identities. Some queer women also identify as bisexual, asexual, or pansexual, as women's feelings of sexual desire and attraction vary greatly mirroring the diversity of women in their own communities (Butler 1990). Many of these identities are explored in later chapters of this text, including Chapters 3, 8, and 9.

The strength of the LGBTQ+ community today is the visible diversity of people with varying sexual orientations and gender identities. Gender, like sexual orientation, is no longer limited to the binary—feminine and masculine—nor is sex limited to female and male. Thus, the universe of women attracted to other women crosses almost, if not all, of the letters of the acronym. When you consider also that sexual identity and gender identity intersect with other identities—race, ethnicity, country of origin, religion, for example—things can get quite complex. These neat little letters can't be so neatly divided for many queer women (Levounis et al. 2012).

Below is a list of definitions connected with the lesbian community (Lesbian, Bisexual, Gay, and Transgender Resource Center 2019; Trans Student Educational Resources 2019; University of California Riverside 2015). These definitions are neither exhaustive nor immutable; asking a woman about her identity term(s) and her interpretations thereof are the only means by which to truly understand the multilayered, nuanced meanings of a given term for any specific individual. The best way to understand what a word means to an individual person is to ask them.

- **ag/aggressive:** Term used by people of color to describe masculine lesbians
- **baby dyke:** Young lesbian who may be early in her acceptance of herself as gay or queer
- **bicurious:** May refer to someone who is gay or straight and also curious about desiring sex and relationships with men or women
- **bi/bisexual:** Refers to people who have sexual attraction and desire for females and males
- **BlaQ/BlaQueer:** People of black/African descent and/or from the African diaspora who recognize their queerness/LGBTQIA identity as a salient identity attached to their Blackness and vice versa
- **boi:** A term used within queer communities of color to refer to sexual orientation, gender, and/or aesthetic among people assigned female at birth. The term is also used by lesbians or genderqueer individuals who express or present themselves in a culturally or stereotypically masculine way.
- **bull dyke:** More of a historical working-class term referring to a masculine or butch lesbian
- **butch:** A lesbian-specific gender identity, originating in women's working-class communities. Associated with the embracing of masculine gender in presentation.
- **cisgender:** When a person's sex assigned at birth aligns with their current gender identity
- **demisexual:** Sexual orientation in which someone feels sexual attraction only to people with whom they have an

emotional bond. Compared with the general population, most demisexuals feel sexual attraction rarely, and some have little to no interest in sexual activity. Considered to be on the asexual spectrum.

- **dyke:** Initially likely used to insult lesbian or gay women
- **femme:** Lesbians or queer women who express or present themselves in a culturally or stereotypically feminine way
- **gay:** Colloquial and affirmative term for homosexual. May refer to men or women, although some women may identify with the term lesbian
- **lesbian:** A woman erotically attracted to women; a sexual identity
- **lipstick lesbian:** A lesbian or queer woman who presents as femme or feminine and passes as heterosexual or straight, which may be upsetting to some femme women
- **pan/pansexual:** A person attracted to all genders on the spectrum
- **queer:** A term for people of marginalized gender identities and sexual orientations who are not cisgender and/or heterosexual. Historically, it was a derogatory term for LGBT people, but it was adopted in the 1990s as a sexual identity by younger gays and lesbians and as a descriptive term for scholarship (queer theory) by academics who favored radical politics or a fluid conception of sexual identity.
- **same gender loving:** Term used by members of the African American/black community to express an alternative sexual orientation
- **stone butch:** A lesbian who may or may not desire sexual reciprocation from her femme sexual partners. Often, a stone butch refers to a lesbian who does not want sexual penetration and/or contact with genitals or breasts
- **stud:** An African American and/or Latina masculine lesbian. Also known as "butch" or "aggressive."

Despite the existence of multiple terminologies, there is still some need to have a dedicated chapter to the "L" among us, whatever we choose to individually call ourselves. This chapter is dedicated to uplifting the voices of the diverse chorus of women who love women. Some of the many identities listed above might be used to describe women in this chapter. Each timbre is distinct and unique, but shared notes are found across the many voices.

# Questions Well-Meaning People Ask

**How does a woman know whether she is a lesbian or if she has just not met the right man yet and may grow out of it?**

Questioning one's sexual orientation is a normal part of identity development during adolescence and for some people into adulthood. To be a supportive friend, family member, or therapist to a woman discovering or questioning her sexual identity, the best thing to do is to support her feelings and awareness but let her come to an identity label on her own. Some studies have suggested that gay women come out to themselves later than do gay men. Others suggest that women simply come out in a different way, discerning affiliation and attraction before having a sexual experience. Same-sex attraction for women is generally not a phase one grows out of over time. However, women can experience fluidity in their sexual identities, with some women who come out as gay later identifying as bisexual or pansexual. Incidentally, some researchers have found that fluidity occurs in men too, although it is spoken about less in the gay male community (Savin-Williams 2017). Musician Hayley Kiyoko recounts her experience (Denton-Hurst 2018):

> I always knew that I liked girls since I was really young. Obviously, everyone has their own personal experience with their family, but eventually my parents were comfortable with it. It just took time. A lot of times, people think it's just a phase. There are also parents who will be accepting of other people, but as soon as it's their kid, it becomes a whole other reality check. That can be hard.

### Don't lesbians really just want to be men?

No, lesbians are women who are attracted to other women. Sexual orientation is not the same as gender identity. If a queer woman has a masculine gender presentation, this is likely not a choice and does not mean that she wants to be male—rather, her gendered behavior and presentation just happen to be more masculine. Lesbians should not be confused with transgender men. Unlike masculine cis women, who are assigned female at birth, transgender men experience their true gender identity as male and may physically transition their bodies to match that identity. Implying that these individuals "want" to be men, however, is also not quite correct and can be as hurtful as suggesting that gay women want to be men (Levitt et al. 2012). Trans men generally feel their male identity as an "is," a deeply felt fact, not a "want to be." Details of transgender identities are explored in Chapter 4.

### If a woman is in a relationship with another woman, doesn't that mean she is a lesbian?

No. Women of different sexual identities may have intimate relationships with other women. Women acting on their feelings of sexual attraction may have relationships with women at different times in their lives. These women may be lesbian, bisexual, pansexual, or heterosexual. At times, women curious about sex with other women may engage in same-sex relationships even though they do not identify as lesbian, queer, bisexual, or pansexual. Some of these women may eventually come out as bisexual or gay, but some may consider themselves straight women who have had gay relationships (Diamond 2009).

### Why do some women use different words for themselves?

The use of sexual orientation identity terms is dynamic and individualized. However, common societal interpretations of these terms exist, and individuals' choice of terms communicates their sense of romantic and sexual self as an extension and reflection of their belonging to various social communities. There is a long list of words women can use to describe themselves, and these words likely mean different things to different people. A list of possible identities you might come across include lesbian, bi, bisexual, queer, pan, pansexual, omnisexual, butch, femme, dyke, bull dyke, baby dyke, softball dyke, non-monosexual, non-mon, BlaQ, gynephillic, gynesexual, lipstick lesbian, same gender loving, stud, aggressive, bicurious, boi, demiromantic, demisexual, high femme, soft butch, stone butch, questioning, and heteroflexible.

### When two women are involved, who initiates the sex? And what do women do in bed anyway?

The idea that women are not sexual beings is a very old stereotype. Women are sexual and assert themselves in relationships with other women. Women may have sex with each other in any of the same ways that women and men have sex. When taking a sexual history with a queer woman patient, a clinician should not assume the patient does or does not engage in any specific activities but should ask. (A common and incorrect stereotype, for example, has been that gay women don't have sex involving penetration or don't enjoy penetration.) It is good practice to ask all patients about sexual history because what the individual calls sex and does in the bedroom can vary from person to person.

**Can you tell that a woman is gay by how she looks?**

Women who love women have a variety of gender identities across the gender spectrum. Some women identify with and embody conventional conceptions of feminine gender expression and may use identity terms that highlight the intersection of their gender expression and sexual orientation (e.g., high femme, lipstick lesbian). Conversely, some women may identify with terms such as butch, stud, or boi, which reflect a queer sexual orientation and more masculine gender expression. Furthermore, gender expression may vary over time (e.g., becoming more masculine or more feminine— even alternating between more feminine and more masculine presentation). Gender expression may also encompass nonbinary gender identities. Women who love women may find varying degrees of femininity, masculinity, and androgyny sexually attractive in prospective intimate partners and may be attracted to partners with similar or dissimilar gender expressions to their own.

**How do I show or tell my gay family member/friend/colleague/student/patient that I support them? I want to be affirming, but I don't know how.**

One important, but easily overlooked, way to show your support is to directly state and emphasize that support, particularly when your family member/friend/colleague/student/patient initially discusses her queer identity with you. Be supportive and open at times when she is emotionally vulnerable, such as when discussing her internal explorations and struggles with her identity, experiences of bias and discrimination, or interpersonal difficulties (e.g., estrangement from family). Statements such as "Thank you for trusting me and sharing this important information with me. I am grateful to be trusted to know more about you" are affirming and can be expanded to introduce follow-up questions (e.g., "I re-spect how important this is and want to make sure I am un-derstanding what you are telling me. Can I ask you a few questions, to help me understand better?"). When questions come from a place of caring and a wish to understand, they are often well received.

It is also important to be sensitive to identifying and creat-ing space for opportunities for a woman to discuss her rela-tionship(s) and involve her partner(s) in social and/or medical engagement. Welcome your loved one, colleague, stu-dent, or client and her intimate partner into the conversation. Be open to having discussions about her intimate partner. It is not helpful or affirming to turn down conversations about her relationship. Recognize the person's intimate partner as such. Ask her how she would like you to address her intimate part-ner. Use respectful language, referring to her date, girlfriend, or intimate partner as an intimate partner, and do not call the person "a friend" or use language that distorts the nature of their relationship. Do not use slang or derogatory language when addressing the person or her intimate partner. In es-sence, be respectful and mindful of the words you use.

## Themes That May Emerge in Therapy

There is no such thing as a single-issue struggle because we do not live single-issue lives.

*Audre Lorde, poet*

### ADDICTION

Although it is generally no longer true that gay bars are the main place where queer people meet, queer people, both men and women, have higher rates of alcohol and drug use disor-ders than the general population. The higher risk is likely due to minority stress—a concept that will be explained multiple times in this text—which generally refers to the stress indi-viduals encounter from being different from the larger popu-lation around them. Histories of sexual and physical trauma, which affect all women, may further increase queer women's risk of addictions. Queer women may benefit from recovery services that address their complete identities and offer sup-port from other queer women.

## BULLYING

Although children, youth, and adult-age lesbians and queer women may experience bullying, gender-nonconforming individuals are at highest risk to become the targets of bullying in elementary, middle, and high school years or by school-age peers. Girls and female youth who dress or present as more masculine, whether or not they later identify as gay, are often targets of bullying. Without a strong support system and healthy self-esteem, these young people or children are vulnerable to verbal and physical violence. Butch lesbians, studs, or bois may be confronted with physical assaults, which may lead them to consider or carry out self-harming or suicidal behavior. Efforts to reduce bullying or threat of violence will provide a more validating environment for women to express their identities.

## COMING OUT

Coming out as a gay woman or lesbian may be a lengthy and complicated process if the youth or woman fears identifying as gay because of stigma. Lesbians and queer youth have been thrown from their homes because of family rejection, and the world continues to be an unsafe place for queer people regardless of where they live. Other young lesbians have experienced support and acceptance, allowing them the opportunity to move through developmental sexual milestones, although the process is rarely a linear one. There is still outside influence from the community, religious organizations, and the media, which can have an effect on a person's identity journey. Furthermore, it is possible for people to come out as gay or lesbian and decide later on that they no longer identify that way—remember that sexual orientation for some can be fluid (Magee and Miller 1997).

It is important to create a safe space for individuals to explore their sexual identity issues and to ask awkward and uncomfortable questions. It is critical that clinicians leave judgment out of the room. Allow people to determine their own sexual orientation and social presentation at their own pace. It is important for people who are coming out to have social supports to help them maintain their emotional health and personal safety. If an individual is worried she will be kicked out of her family and home, listen to her and honor her fears until it is clear that she is in a safe place at home or elsewhere. Too many LGBTQ+ young people are disowned by their families and become homeless overnight.

Clinicians should be mindful that people who appear to be knowledgeable about the LGBTQ+ community might also need help with the coming out process. Even lesbian or queer-identified moms might need help with their children in the coming out process. Some parents in their supportive enthusiasm have outed their children on social media, leaving children and young people in an awkward and vulnerable position. Children and youth should talk with their supportive parents and family members about the different ways to come out. Communication is key. There are pros and cons in every situation, and children and youth need time to reflect on these issues rather than impulsively coming out to their larger communities.

## COMING OUT AROUND THE WORLD

The experience of coming out as a lesbian in countries outside of the United States lies on a spectrum of acceptance through imprisonment and risk of death by death penalty. Even in the United States, LGBTQ+ people do not have equal civil rights to their straight counterparts. Individual liberties can differ greatly depending on geographic location. Queer people can lose their jobs, homes, access to medical care, or parental rights despite recent civil rights progress. Be mindful of people from other countries who have fled their homelands out of fear of persecution. Some patients may need help with asylum because returning to their countries of birth could mean imprisonment or death.

## DEATH AND DYING

End-of-life issues for lesbian and queer women may be simple or more complicated depending on the level of pre-preparation that has been done legally. Some lesbians choose to legally outline their rights and specifications for medical treatment as well as for what they own. Death-related concerns can become more complicated depending on the degree of family support and acceptance, as well as the strength of friendships and other social supports involved in the process. Lesbians with strong community and family supports who lose their lesbian spouse or intimate partner may live more satisfying or positive lives versus spending their lives in isolation.

Those with fewer supports are at an increased risk for suicide. Bereavement counseling and support groups are important resources for survivors. When working with patients who are either dying or have lost a loved one, be mindful of their social network and supports.

## FAMILY

Lesbians have built families with varying degrees of biological family members versus chosen family members. Queer women have been having children as long as there have been people. Whether or not they have been out about their identities during this process is another story. We know that gay and lesbian parents have children who are no different from the children of heterosexual parents.

Lesbians or queer women bring children to their relationships in a variety of ways. Some women have children together using sperm from chosen donors. Some women come out later in life after having had children from heterosexual relationships. Other women choose to have children by becoming foster parents or through adoption. Laws around parental rights may differ from state to state. Patients should be encouraged to be aware of the legal aspects regarding their children. It is also important for queer parents to be aware that their struggles with their children are typically not due to the parent's queer identities. Some queer mothers who have troubled children might blame their queer identity as the cause; however, all parents have some difficulties with their children, and queer parents should be reminded that this is true for them, just as for any other parent. It is important for clinicians to be aware how the many different facets of a person's identity can affect an already complicated parent-child relationship.

## INTERPERSONAL VIOLENCE

Gay women and lesbians, just like any person, can act in violent ways—emotionally, verbally, physically, and sexually. Whether they are more feminine, more masculine, or somewhere in between, women can be both the victim or perpetrator of violence in intimate relationships. Similar to straight peers who batter, gay women are brought up in families where domestic abuse occurs, and individuals may experience the violence directly or by witnessing it. Be aware of your own assumptions around women in relationships and understand that there are many ways in which violence can manifest.

## LEGAL ISSUES

The U.S. Supreme Court guaranteed same-sex couples the fundamental right to marry in *Obergefell v. Hodges* in 2015, but, despite the new freedoms, many queer couples who have openly married have suffered consequences due to their expressions of love. Some have found themselves legally unemployed through job termination, homeless after being kicked out of their housing by homophobic landlords, or faced with finding new health providers because their doctors don't feel they are morally obligated to treat queer people. Political climates can vary greatly, and queer women unfortunately have to consider potential consequences they might face due to their sexual identity. Because of confidentiality, a mental health provider's office might be the only place a queer woman feels safe expressing herself and asking questions about her health.

## MINORITY STRESS

Ilan Meyer, Ph.D., developed a model of stress and illness in minority populations that demonstrates that discrimination and prejudice have an additive effect on minority individuals at the intersection of their sexual orientation, race, ethnicity, and gender identities (Meyer 2003). Dr. Meyer's research has also demonstrated that sexual minority individuals with multiple minority identities have poorer health and mental health outcomes due to these additive effects. Research using the minority stress model has been effective in demonstrating the impact of social stressors on increasing risk for addiction, homelessness, unemployment, isolation, sexual violence, interpersonal violence, suicide, and homicide. In the past, some people might have blamed a person's identity as the cause of their increased stressors. This turned out to be true, but not in the way imagined. Having a minority status in a larger homogenous community is likely the cause. If minority people were surrounded by people who were like them, they likely would not face these medical and mental health disparities.

## RELIGION AND SPIRITUALITY

Despite a sordid history of religious nonacceptance, queer people are finding many more supportive religious groups today. Even so, many gay and lesbian women who value their religious life and community continue to experience loss of church and other religious communities because of their identities. This loss may be a particularly devastating experience for some individuals and families who have grown up within a tight-knit religious community. Finding themselves rejected by their community may be as or more harmful than losing family. When meeting with an individual who is working through these loss issues, you must first understand the seriousness of this loss in the person's mind and then support them through their grief process. Some religious groups are more judgmental or harsh than others. Levels of prejudice can vary widely within religions that have otherwise homogenous ideologies. Some religions have been guilty of outright abusive behavior toward queer women. Religion can often be thought of as another support network that may need attention to ensure a person's safety. Gaychurch.org is a website helpful to those in need of finding a religious home.

## SAME-SEX PARENTING

Same-sex parents are visible today in schools in larger numbers than ever before. Same-sex parents deserve the same respect from teachers and administrators given to their heterosexual counterparts. It is important for schools to have safe spaces for parents and children and be mindful that a parent's sexual identity may create unique situations depending on the overall acceptance level of the community.

Queer parents will often deal with their own set of challenges. As their child ages, they will likely need to come out all over again to a new set of people—teachers, day care providers, pediatricians. Helping parents find groups of same-sex parents and their allies may be the most effective way to support parents and their children. Connecting parents to support such as COLAGE (www.colage.org) and Family Equality (www.familyequality.org), as well as other resources, may be helpful.

## SUICIDE

Rates of suicide and suicidal behavior have long been identified as being significantly higher in queer people than straight peers. LGB youth ages 10–24 years have suicidal ideation about three times as often as heterosexual peers (Centers for Disease Control and Prevention 2016). This is largely believed to be likely due to minority stress, as mentioned previously. Suicidal behavior is increased in gay female youth, and clinicians should be mindful of this when doing suicide assessments or working with patients in crisis (Haas et al. 2011).

## WOMEN OF COLOR

Everything previously said about risk factors and minority stress needs to take into account that queer women of color will experience increased doses of stigma and harm or even more, depending on their intersecting identities (National Center for Health Statistics 2012). The data on black women being at increased risk for pregnancy complications and loss, regardless of their socioeconomic status and access to health care, show that minority stress is expressed in a variety of ways. Queer ethnic minority women face increased stigma, discrimination, and stress burden. They may also have a harder time building a support network. Women of color may have a more difficult time finding community within lesbian social circles and organizations, which will likely be majority white and may feel unwelcoming to women of color. When working with queer women of color, consider how a woman's race may affect her current life stressors and be open to conversations about race.

# Conclusion

Lesbian or gay women are a diverse group who have a range of ways in which they identify and express themselves romantically. Clinicians can provide better care by approaching each case individually and not placing queer women into boxes. Given the intersectionality of identity, gender, and other factors such as ethnicity, lesbian or gay women face many stressors that could have an impact on their mental health, highlighting the need for attention to be placed on the whole person.

# FIVE TAKE-HOME POINTS

- Women's sexual orientation and identity are often complex and can vary from individual to individual.

- The cultural landscape for queer women continues to change. The best way to keep up is to be open to asking friends, family, and patients about their experiences.

- Despite increased visibility and acceptance, lesbians continue to face discrimination and risks due to minority stress.

- Try to consider queer women's identities as multidimensional, taking into account all aspects of their self when working with them from a clinical standpoint.

- When possible, make space for queer women to talk about their lives by creating an environment that is judgment free.

## Resources

Association of American Medical Colleges: Sexual and gender minority health resources. Washington, DC, Association of American Medical Colleges, 2019. Available at: www.aamc.org/initiatives/diversity/lgbthealthresources
Association of LGBTQ Psychiatrists: www.aglp.org
International Lesbian, Gay, Bisexual, Trans and Intersex Association: https://ilga.org
National LGBT Health Education Center: www.lgbthealth education.org

## References

Butler J: Gender Trouble: Feminism and the Subversion of Identity. London, Routledge, 1990
Centers for Disease Control and Prevention: Sexual Identity, Sex of Sexual Contacts, and Health-Risk Behaviors Among Students in Grades 9-12: Youth Risk Behavior Surveillance. Atlanta, GA: U.S. Department of Health and Human Services, 2016

Denton-Hurst T: How Hayley Kiyoko lived her truth and became the "queen savior" of pop. San Francisco, CA, PopSugar, June 21, 2018. Available at: www.popsugar.com/entertainment/Hayley-Kiyoko-LGBTQ-Pride-Month-Interview-44888006. Accessed January 23, 2020.

Diamond LM: Sexual Fluidity: Understanding Women's Love and Desire. Cambridge, MA, Harvard University Press, 2009

Haas AP, Eliason M, Mays VM, et al: Suicide and suicide risk in lesbian, gay, bisexual, and transgender populations: review and recommendations. J Homosex 58(1):10–51, 2011 21213174

Lesbian, Bisexual, Gay, and Transgender Resource Center: LGBTQA+ glossary. East Lansing, Michigan State University, 2019. Available at: http://lbgtrc.msu.edu/educational-resources/glossary-of-lgbtq-terms. Accessed January 28, 2020.

Levitt HM, Puckett JA, Ippolito MR, Horne SG: Sexual minority women's gender identity and expression: challenges and supports. J Lesbian Stud 16(2):153–176, 2012 22455340

Levounis P, Drescher J, Barber ME: The LGBT Casebook. Washington, DC, American Psychiatric Publishing, 2012

Magee M, Miller DC: Lesbian Lives: Psychoanalytic Narratives Old and New. Hillsdale, NJ, Analytic Press, 1997

Meyer IH: Prejudice, social stress, and mental health in lesbian, gay, and bisexual populations: conceptual issues and research evidence. Psychol Bull 129(5):674–697, 2003 12956539

National Center for Health Statistics: Special feature on socioeconomic status and health, in Health, United States, 2011. Hyattsville, MD, National Center for Health Statistics, 2012. Available at: www.cdc.gov/nchs/hus/contents2011.htm. Accessed February 25, 2020.

Savin-Williams RC: Mostly Straight: Sexual Fluidity Among Men. Cambridge, MA, Harvard University Press, 2017

Trans Student Educational Resources: LGBTQ+ definitions. Trans Student Educational Resources, 2019. Available at: www.transstudent.org/definitions. Accessed January 28

University of California Riverside: LGBT terminology. Riverside University of California Riverside, 2015. Available at: http://students673.ucr.edu/docsserver/lgbt/terminology.pdf. Accessed January 28.

# Chapter 2

# Gay

## The G in LGBTQ$^2$IAPA

AHMAD A. MOHAMMAD, M.D.
ERIC YARBROUGH, M.D.

Why is it that, as a culture, we are more comfortable seeing two men holding guns, than holding hands?

*Ernest Gaines*

## Psychological and Cultural Context

Gay men and gay culture are vast and diverse topics that have been written about in numerous volumes throughout human history. Attempting to condense this subject into one chapter requires touching superficially on the most relevant subjects that pertain to medical and mental health professionals. Although we have attempted to condense this material, we hope that this brief overview will encourage further exploration of subtopics covered in this chapter. Suggestions for further reading will be given at the end of the chapter.

Gay men have existed as long as people have existed. Although some cultures (e.g., ancient Greece) have been more accepting of same-sex practices, throughout history the majority of cultures have kept gay men in the shadows of civilization. Even today, engaging in same-sex relationships can lead to punishment by death in many countries.

The main trouble in understanding gay men is first identifying what the term *gay* refers to. Gay could refer to men who have sex with men, but those same men may or may not self-identify as gay. A gay identity does not imply that someone is having sex with men or that they are even having sex. In addition, many men who identify as straight engage in same-sex relationships.

To further expand on the complex identity of being gay, the concept of gender factors in as well. There are a variety of gender identities (including transgender and gender nonbinary) and gender presentations, each of which might describe an individual who identifies as gay. Many women who engage in same-sex relationships also refer to themselves as gay. Using the term gay does not directly correlate to a person who was assigned male at birth and engages in same-sex sexual relationships. It is important to see each individual as just that, an individual. An ongoing focus throughout this book is not making assumptions and approaching each person with open-minded curiosity. Given that most of the other identities related to the term gay are covered elsewhere in this book, for the rest of this chapter we focus on cis gay men as largely understood by western culture. Below is a broad overview of terms used in gay culture.

- **baby gay:** A newly out or recently self-identified gay individual
- **bareback:** Sexual intercourse without a condom
- **BDSM:** This acronym stands for bondage and sadomasochism and is part of a sexual kink subculture found in all sexualities
- **bear:** Subculture in the gay community; typically, a bear is a larger, hairy man
- **beard:** Often used to describe ways a man might hide himself to avoid being perceived as gay (e.g., having a wife)
- **bottom:** The receptive partner during anal sex
- **breeding/seeding:** When one sexual partner ejaculates into the other while having bareback sex
- **bug chaser:** An HIV-negative man who has unprotected receptive sex with HIV-positive men in the hope of seroconversion
- **butch:** A man who identifies as possessing traditionally masculine traits. Often related to stereotypically straight male identifiers such as voice, dress, behavior, and activities. Similar to masc.
- **catcher:** The receptive partner during anal sex. This is an older term similar to bottom.
- **cisgender:** When a person's sex assigned at birth aligns with their current gender identity

- **clean:** A derogatory term in gay slang that means someone is HIV negative
- **cruising:** A gay culture phenomenon used to describe the act of seeking gay sexual encounters through eye contact and body language
- **discreet:** A term used when a man wants to have sex with a man but wants to keep it a secret
- **dom:** A shortened version of *dominant*, referring to the dominant partner in a relationship or during sexual intercourse
- **down low (DL):** A man (sometimes associated with African American men) who has sex with men but keeps it a secret; may or may not identify as gay
- **drag:** When men dress up in women's clothing, usually for entertainment or cultural purposes
- **faggot:** A derogatory term used to describe gay men that is now sometimes used by gay men in an endearing way
- **fairy:** A previously derogatory term referring to a gay man that has been reclaimed by the gay community
- **femme:** A man who identifies as possessing traditionally feminine traits, often related to stereotypically gay male identifiers such as effeminate voice, dress, behavior, and/or activities
- **fisting:** A sexual act in which one partner inserts a hand into the other partner's anus
- **friend of Dorothy:** Term referring to Dorothy from *The Wizard of Oz* (with an association to the song "Somewhere Over the Rainbow"), used to describe a gay man
- **gay:** An umbrella term that generally refers to men who are attracted to other men
- **gayborhood:** A neighborhood with a high concentration of gay people, serving as an important safe space for members of the community
- **gold star:** A gay man who has never had sex with a female
- **heteroflexible:** Refers to a straight-identifying man who occasionally has sex with men
- **homophobia:** Fear, prejudice, and/or hatred toward anything related to homosexuality
- **homosexual:** A person who is sexually attracted to someone of the same sex. The term can also be used to describe sex or events that happen with gay men.
- **in the closet (closeted):** Refers to someone who is gay but has not told anyone or has not been involved with the larger gay community

- **internalized homophobia:** Self-stigma generated by the internalization of societal negativity and prejudice toward and discrimination against homosexuality
- **kiki:** A relatively new term to refer to gay men gathering to talk and/or gossip
- **kink:** Sexual activity that is outside the realm of typical oral or anal sex (e.g., fisting)
- **looking:** Seeking casual sexual encounters; similar to cruising
- **masc:** A man who identifies as possessing traditionally masculine traits. Often related to stereotypically straight male identifiers such as voice, dress, behavior, and activities
- **MSM:** Men who have sex with men
- **outing:** Telling others that an individual is gay, thus bringing that person out of the closet. It is generally thought to be a negative act.
- **party and play (PNP):** A term referring to gay men who are open to using substances (e.g., crystal meth) during sex
- **pig:** A gay man who wants to be involved with kinkier sexual activity (e.g., breeding)
- **pink triangle:** A reclaimed symbol from Nazi Germany that was used to identify gay citizens
- **pitcher:** The penetrative/insertive partner during anal sex. This is an older term similar to top
- **poppers:** Alkyl or amyl nitrites in vials from which fumes of the liquid are often inhaled recreationally at clubs or bars and before sex. Although initially used to treat angina, this chemical acts as a vasodilator, causing increased heart rate and blood flow, which creates a "head rush" or euphoria. Furthermore, the smooth muscle relaxant effect, including the anal sphincter, can facilitate anal sex.
- **poz:** A slang term for someone who is HIV positive
- **pride:** A complex self-identity acceptance and expression used to communicate that a person is happy about and proud of being gay
- **puppy play:** A subculture within the gay community that involves role-play using costumes resembling puppies or dogs
- **queen:** Term used to describe a gay man; can be positive if used by a friend. Within the gay community, it can be a term of endearment.
- **queer:** A reclaimed word that used to be derogatory but now can be used to mean anyone in the LGBTQ spectrum
- **rimming:** An oral-anal sex act

During the twentieth century, gay culture and identities started to become more common. Gay bars located in major cities, just like today, provided gay men the chance to meet others who were like themselves. It was a place for them to be surrounded by others and express their authentic selves.

One pivotal moment in gay history occurred in 1969 at the Stonewall Inn, a local gay bar in New York City. This bar, like so many other gay bars around the city and the world, was often raided by police, and patrons were arrested for perverse behavior. Following in the energy created by the civil rights movement over the previous 20 years, on the day that Judy Garland (a popular gay icon; see "friend of Dorothy" in the previous section) died, gay and gender-diverse patrons fought back against the police—starting the Stonewall Riots. This marked the birth of what would become the gay civil rights movement. Free love, diversity, and identity would start to blossom for the gay culture in the 1970s in the United States.

The positive movements forward, however, would take a pivotal turn in the early 1980s with the emergence of the HIV/AIDS epidemic. Although anyone can contract HIV, gay men were particularly affected because of sexual relationships that involved anal sex. For this reason, many people thought AIDS was a "gay disease," and it was initially named GRID (gay-related immune deficiency). Scores of gay men died during this time, and friendships and families were torn apart. Thousands of deaths occurred over many years, leading to protests before effective treatment was finally researched. Many of the scars and trauma created from the loss of life during this time still reside today in the older gay population who survived the plague. The fear created by HIV/AIDS also lingers within the younger gay community, which puts up barriers in physical relationships between gay men.

HIV/AIDS and safe sex practice became better understood in last decade of the twentieth century. The emergence of antiretroviral medications also decreased infection rates. Although HIV/AIDS left a permanent impact on the gay community, same-sex relationships were still flourishing, and gay culture turned its sights to basic human rights—the ability to get married and have children. Although it is certainly not universal in the community, many gay men want to have the option to have a spouse and children like the rest of society. Legal battles ensued, and in 2004 Massachusetts became the first state to legalize same-sex marriage (*Goodridge v. Department of Public Health*). State-by-state legal battles culminated in 2015 with the Supreme Court ruling on *Obergefell v. Hodges* that legalized same-sex marriage.

Although the United States and some other countries around the world have legalized same-sex marriage and provided gay people with adoption rights, these freedoms are still not present universally around the world. Furthermore, these civil rights victories continue to be challenged by people who oppose sexual orientation diversity, such as in *Masterpiece Cakeshop v. Colorado Civil Rights Commission* (2018).

## PSYCHOLOGICAL OVERVIEW

The development of gay men throughout their lifespan is similar in some ways to that of straight people, but it goes without question that individuals with a gay identity experience unique stressors not present in the heterosexual world. Although research on gay development exists, this research suffers from the aforementioned complexity of gay identity. It is difficult to study gay men because it is still not clear who gay men are. Some people use the term "men who have sex with men" in an attempt to encompass same-sex relationships regardless of identity. Although research efforts are improving, gay men, like all queer people, are poorly understood and are underrepresented in scientific research.

Many gay men report the sense of feeling different throughout childhood. Some discover this uniqueness early on, whereas for others it might take a lifetime. Some gay men are effeminate by societal norms, and those who are effeminate at a young age are often the target of harassment, bullying, and abuse. As a result, many gay men spend a great deal of energy attempting to hide their sexual orientation so as not to bring on unwanted and negative attention. The common phenomenon of the *false self* can develop (Drescher 2001), putting gay men in the position of projecting an outward heterosexual identify while their true self (the one with same-sex feelings) is hidden away. This dual-role identity can become difficult to tease apart in psychotherapy, and many gay men require encouragement and validation to discover their core identity.

Gay men are also exposed to the thoughts and views of the societies in which they are raised. Because the majority of society has negative views of homosexuality, gay men internalize those views after being exposed to them by their family, religion, and community. These internalized negative views are generally understood to be the reason for gay men's higher rates of depression, anxiety, substance use, and suicide (Meyer 2003). The term for this is *internalized homophobia,* and the concept is well known among clinicians who work with people of diverse sexual orientations. In addition, because everyone is exposed to homophobic thoughts and ideas, all of us have some level of internalized homophobia. Medical and mental health providers must be mindful of this when working with gay men.

Coming out can be a difficult time for gay men. The term *coming out* refers to the developmental period when individuals discover, understand, and communicate their same-sex attraction to themselves and other people in their lives. This process can happen at any stage of life from adolescence to old age. Many who come out find the process stressful, and this time can lead to increased symptomatology. Mood lability, impulsivity, suicidal thoughts—often correlated with a host of other psychiatric conditions—can occur when someone is coming out. A lack of understanding of this process can lead to misdiagnosis and excess treatment with some individuals.

## Questions Well-Meaning People Ask

### What does it mean to be gay?

To answer this question, it is important to understand the difference between sexual orientation, sexual identity, and sexual behavior. Although all are interconnected, they may not always parallel the common conceptualization of the term *gay,* and each aspect is different to each individual person. Briefly, gay sexual orientation is a pattern of emotional, sexual, and/or romantic feelings for members of the same sex or gender identity. This is distinct from gender identity or gender expression. Sexual identity refers to one's perception of self and can involve identity components unrelated to sexuality. Sexual behavior refers to sexual activity or conduct. A man who experiences sexual attraction to other men and may engage in sex with men might identify as gay but might also identify as bisexual or straight. These concepts should be understood as fluid rather than discrete entities, and it is often better to give people space for self-identification.

### Is being gay a choice?

No, being gay is not a choice, the same way being straight is not a choice. There has not been conclusive evidence that any set of factors influences sexual orientation, and there is no significant amount of evidence to identify a specific reason—developmental, genetic, hormonal, and/or social—that someone is gay. Although it is clear that the effects of nature and nurture on sexual orientation are complex, sexual orientation is not a choice.

## How do gay men know they are gay?

Many gay men recall feeling different early in adolescence, a theme that continues throughout their sexual development. This realized differentness can be related to several reasons, including homoerotic interests or attractions, gender atypical behavior, or even shame generated by heteronormative nonconformity. Often, gay men are aware of their orientation before having sexual experiences and may engage in sexual behavior only after coming to terms with their sexuality. It takes time, introspection, and exploration to understand those feelings, and these developmental milestones are different for each person.

## Could being gay be just a phase?

Some people, as seen in Chapter 6, "Questioning," may be in a part of their life in which they do not really know how to define their sexual orientation. They think they might be gay but are still confused about their feelings. This might be due to societal or family pressure to identify as heterosexual. They might also have more bisexual or pansexual feelings and do not feel that the term gay encompasses their sexual orientation experience. Sexual orientation is also somewhat fluid, so people can move in and out of phases in their life when they might be more attracted to particular genders or no gender at all. If someone comes out to you as gay, however, they should be taken seriously. Only with support and affirmation can people be free to figure out who they are without judgment.

## Is it possible for gay men to change their sexual orientation?

This topic has been and remains quite controversial. Some men claim they have been "cured" and changed their sexual orientation from gay to straight. This is unlikely because sexual orientation is not a choice and develops over time. Rather, it is plausible for an individual to have a natural change in sexual desires given the fluidity of sexual orientation and attraction. Furthermore, forced treatment attempts, including reparative or conversion therapy—attempting to change a person's sexual orientation from gay to straight—are not only ineffective but also extremely risky and traumatic. They can even lead to suicide. These attempts have been denounced by the medical community for putting victims at risk for developing several debilitating and self-destructive conditions. Because of this, the practice of conversion therapy is becoming illegal in many states.

**Can I tell if someone is gay just by looking at them?**

No. Gay men are a diverse group of individuals spanning all age groups, socioeconomic backgrounds, races, cultures, and religions and are found in every single part of the world. Inferences about orientation often arise from inaccurate stereotypes that are propagated and reinforced by society and the media. Although some gay men may fit certain cultural traits associated with a gay identity, others do not. Assuming sexual orientation on the basis of any number of attributes such as appearance/dress, behavior, gender norms, or even career choices is not possible. Although the inferences may seem harmless, they unfortunately serve to victimize both the gay men who may or may not fit those stereotypes and non-gay men who do. At the same time, they legitimize inaccurate perceptions of gay men and reinforce prejudice and oppression.

**What does it mean to "come out," and why is it important?**

Coming out, or *coming out of the closet*, refers to disclosing sexual minority status to others. It is a lifelong process occurring innumerable times throughout one's life. Although on the surface, coming out seems as simple as telling someone you are gay, it is much more complex. Coming out requires self-discovery and integration of dissociated traits of self. Only with validation and space can people feel free to express their sexual orientation how they see fit. Disclosing one's sexual identity to others is often an active event complicated further by social, cultural, and/or religious dimensions. This rite of passage is unique and multifaceted for each person.

**Do gay men care about religion?**

Just as with anyone else, religion may or may not be important to a gay man. The relationship between gay men and religion can be complicated. Many people and institutions have used religion as a way to deny gay people civil rights, to make homosexuality illegal, and even to punish gay men with death. Religion can be a healthy or unhealthy addition to a person's life. Some gay men find comfort and community in religion, and the complex relationship each person has with religion should be explored when individuals are in a therapeutic setting.

**Are gay men more sexual or promiscuous?**

Like heterosexuals, some gay men are more sexual or promiscuous, whereas others are not. Sexual desire, behavior, and expression are complex and vary for each person, and they are not predicted by sexual orientation. Some would say that gay men have more freedom to express themselves than do heterosexuals. Having been denied civil rights such as marriage, until recently, gay men were not bound by traditional views of marriage and monogamy. Many gay men are monogamous with their partners, but sexual freedom and expression has often been associated with gay culture as a whole.

**Is HIV/AIDS a gay-related disease?**

No. Early in the disease history while researchers were trying to understand the cause, it was noted that HIV was disproportionately affecting gay men, and thus the resulting disease was erroneously coined gay-related immune deficiency. Although gay men are disproportionately affected by HIV, it is important to note that infections are determined not by sexual orientation but rather by sexual behavior. Unprotected receptive anal sex carries the highest risk for acquiring the infection, and this includes people who do not identify as gay. Although a significant number of heterosexuals engage in anal sex (and other forms of unprotected sex), this risk was previously ignored by people shaping public health policy.

**Does the introduction of PrEP enable MSM to engage in high-risk sexual behavior?**

Changes in sexual behavior in people taking pre-exposure prophylaxis (PrEP) is still under study, but to date there has been no substantive evidence of increased risk-taking among PrEP users. However, gay men are more cautious than heterosexuals about the risks associated with sexual behavior and are more likely to use condoms specifically for prevention of sexually transmitted diseases. The reality is there are many reasons why someone seeks PrEP including serodiscordance (in which one partner is HIV positive and the other is not), reduction in anxiety about HIV, preventing disease, and enabling sexual pleasure.

**How are gay men as parents?**

Gay men are as fit as parents as heterosexual people, and their children fare just as well as children raised by heterosexual families. This is evidenced across multiple metrics (Crowl et al. 2008), and virtually all major health organizations that deal with issues related to parenting and childcare (e.g., American Psychiatric Association, American Psychological Association, American Academy of Pediatrics) have issued statements supporting parenting rights of LGBTQ+ individuals. Furthermore, there is no empirical evidence to suggest gay men would harm their children or that their sexual orientation might influence a child's sexual identity development.

**Are gay men trying to recruit others to be gay?**

No. Providing inclusive environments is a major tenet of gay culture, and being supportive of people who might be confused or trying to understand their sexual identity is just as critical. With that comes the understanding that everyone has a right to be themselves, including straight people. Established gay men may serve in a mentoring or fostering role, thereby creating a safe space, especially for those at less mature states of sexual identity development. Because sexuality is not a choice and develops over time, the mentee is often someone who is gay and is in the process of coming out. Unfortunately, the myth of a recruiting strategy or "gay agenda" often serves to vilify gay people, encouraging continued persecution, discrimination, and marginalization in multiple aspects of gay people's lives. There are likely still many gay people who are in the closet and have yet to come out because of fear of rejection and stigmatization. Having an open and supportive environment simply provides a space to come out for gay people who were already there in the first place.

**Can't gay men just decide not to have sex, even if they are attracted to men?**

This suggestion could be imposed on any group of people, but it is simply unrealistic. Furthermore, some would argue that forcing gays to choose celibacy and forcing suppression of a deeply intrinsic part of themselves is really just another form of conversion therapy. Although advocating that gay men abstain entirely from gay sex may not be seeking a "cure" in the same way, it still manages to seek a cure for sexual behavior that is prevalent in heterosexual relationships. It vilifies and singles out gay men for the deeply innate human desire for sexual pleasure, for the rest of their lives, in a way that does not apply to heterosexual people. Even in societies where abstaining from sex until marriage is the idealized norm, gay men do not have this option. However, some gay men do choose to be celibate as a way to reconcile their faith with their same-sex attractions. Although this may bring some of those men happiness, others may wonder if this suppression is a manifestation of internalized homophobia.

## Do gay marriages work out long term?

Many do and many do not. When gay people have access to marriage, their marriages are as stable as heterosexual marriages. It has only been in the past few years that gay men have been allowed to legally marry in the United States, and because of this recent change there has been little research on the longevity of same-sex marriage. There are studies that indicate gay marriages may be more stable than heterosexual marriages (e.g., Joyner et al., 2017) for several reasons—for instance, the adversity from external pressures that couples must overcome may strengthen the bond between them. The point is that relationships and marriage are complicated regardless of sexual orientation, and as with other population groups, there are many variables involved in maintaining them.

## Are gay men more prone to mental illness and substance use?

Like other marginalized groups, gay men tend to suffer higher rates of mental illness and substance use. However, this susceptibility is not thought to be caused by homosexuality itself; rather, it is at least partly explained by the minority stress model, as discussed in Chapter 1, "Lesbian." Gay men have historically had much hostility and violence directed at them and in many parts of the world continue to face stigma, discrimination, and other institutionalized means of oppression. With homosexuality being pathologized not only in the public sphere but even within medicine, and with limited access to appropriate care and interventions, it is not surprising that LGBTQ+ people would experience higher rates of mental illnesses than the general population.

### Now that gay men can get married, can they still say they are oppressed?

Although significant strides have been made to allow same-sex couples marriage equality, there is still a long way to go. Although same-sex marriages are legal in the United States, there continue to be legal and societal attacks on the right of two men (or two women) to marry, which dehumanizes the LGBTQ+ community. Furthermore, denial of marriage equality is only one facet of oppression in a long history of injustice toward gay people. In some countries, gay men do not have the same legal protections afforded to heterosexual people, such as anti-discrimination laws, and in other places being gay can cost them their lives.

### What is internalized homophobia?

Internalized homophobia is the internalization of negative societal or community attitudes toward homosexuality, leading to self-stigma and prejudice toward other homosexuals. The degree to which a person experiences internalized homophobia is dependent on multiple factors, including the level of social hostility toward the LGBTQ+ community, heteronormative cultural expectations, and the person's own management of intrapsychic conflict. Internalized homophobia can be conscious or unconscious and can affect a person in varying degrees. It can have far-reaching consequences, causing gay men to conform to heteronormativity to distance themselves from the LGBTQ+ community as a defense mechanism.

### Why is there special training focused on gay men in health care?

Men who have sex with men and are younger than age 25, especially those from a racial or ethnic minority group, account for a disproportionate number of HIV diagnoses. LGBTQ+ youth have higher rates of suicidal ideation and suicide attempts (Mustanski et al. 2010). Risk factors, such as harassment, victimization, and violence, for mental health problems and substance use are higher for LGBTQ+ youth than for their heterosexual peers. Additional risk factors, including smoking, alcohol use, substance use, and homelessness may be more prevalent in LGBTQ+ youth populations. LGBTQ+

people—transgender people in particular—face disproportionately high rates of mental illness, HIV, unemployment, poverty, and harassment. A poll conducted by NPR, the Robert Wood Johnson Foundation, and the Harvard T.H. Chan School of Public Health found that one in five LGBTQ adults has avoided medical care because of fear of discrimination (NPR et al. 2017). According to the Kaiser Family Foundation, approximately half of all gay and bisexual men have never discussed their sexual orientation with a physician (Hamel et al. 2014). Overlooking this facet of patients' identities can have detrimental consequences to their health.

# Themes That May Emerge in Therapy

## CHILDHOOD AND ADOLESCENCE

Although many gay adults recall feeling or knowing that they were "different" early on, others may not encounter this feeling or may not understand it until later in life. Sometimes, gay adolescents or adults may report that they "always knew" they were gay, but this is often related to a display of atypical gender behavior or atypical traits, such as effeminate demeanor, crossdressing, or playing with girls' toys. These children may face some level of insult and bullying from their family or peers, as well as negative reinforcement from society, leading to feelings of guilt, shame, and poor self-esteem.

However, it must be noted that all children experiment as they begin to understand and develop their identities, and these phases do not necessarily mean a child is gay or straight. Boys who "act like girls," oppose gender-typical roles, or show same-sex affection are not necessarily gay, although many might be. Thus, it is important to avoid conflating gender behavior and sexual orientation. The best practice is to wait to see how a child progresses over time and give them space for self-expression. To avoid suppressing children's developing identities, causing them to feel marginalized and ultimately to experience internalized homophobia, it is better to support children and adolescents for who they are.

For the clinician, it is important to recognize that atypical teens may not have anyone to talk with about their experiences and that they need a safe space to process their feelings. Creating a welcoming and nonjudgmental space for these patients, being open to answering questions, and making inclusive statements will minimize distress and encourage rapport. Ensuring them that everyone has a different experience will allow patients to feel comfortable exploring their identities and prevent ostracism.

## COMING OUT

Simply put, *coming out* or *coming out of the closet* describes a lifelong ongoing process or rite of passage in which a gay person becomes aware of, acknowledges, and discloses their sexual identity. Multiple models for this process exist, and they serve to capture a general theme of progressive subjective experiences, which are much more complex than outlined here. It is important to note that stages may not occur sequentially, some stages may not occur at all, and people may revisit stages or experience them simultaneously (Horowitz and Newcomb 2002). In general, coming out involves coming out to self and coming out to others. Coming out to self involves the following stages (Eckstrand and Ehrenfeld 2016; Rosario et al. 2006):

- Awareness of heterosexual incongruence
- Exploration of an unfolding gay identity
- Integration and consolidation of dissociated aspects of self

Heterosexual incongruence encompasses an awareness of differentness, same-sex attraction and fantasies, and questioning one's sexual identity. During exploration, both social and sexual experimentation may be involved, which requires unlearning the expectations of heteronormative identity while learning the gay culture one is entering (Levounis et al. 2012). Identity integration allows one to accept and manage a gay identity, resolving the negative attitudes of internalized homophobia, and integrating intrapersonal traits beyond sexual identity (Rosario et al. 2006). This consolidation is often described as the pivotal moment of coming to terms with being gay.

Coming out is a shared cultural experience unique to LGBTQ+ people, but it is also a variable and uniquely individualized experience given the heterogeneity of factors involved. These factors include personality traits, individual psychosocial development, cultural and family dynamics, and environmental context. Because of the variability of these components, the coming-out process occurs on different time lines depending on the person. There is no one correct way to come out.

## SEX

Sex and the gay community have changed dramatically over the past 50 years. Until recently, gay men were more a part of fringe society. If a gay man wanted to meet another gay man, he had to be part of the subculture and know where gay men would congregate. Sometimes this would be in a particular bar, park, or highway rest area. Knowing where to meet other gay men was underground secret knowledge.

Gay bars became a staple meeting place in many cities, and this still is true in many places. It became common for these gay bars to be raided by police, and the men inside were arrested. Only after the Stonewall Riots and the start of the gay civil rights movement did this start to change. The gay civil rights movement made dramatic changes to the way gay people are perceived by the larger public, but the movement veered off course with the emergency of HIV (see subsection "HIV").

Today, gay men have access to a score of online apps that provide easy avenues to finding a sexual partner. These apps are tailored to specific desires gay men might have. As with many aspect of gay culture, however, online apps come with both pros and cons. Although they provide a level of sexual freedom and expression, online apps also make room for discrimination and prejudice. Gay men, like anyone else, can be racist and even homophobic. Apps that provide some level of anonymity can make it easy for those with negative views to express themselves.

One of the more complicated things about gay sex is understanding precisely what that term means. Although many people might think that gay sex refers only to anal sex, there are wide opinions about what constitutes sexual activity. Some might consider kissing to be sexual activity, and others might say that anal sex is not necessarily sex unless it includes a romantic feeling.

One positive aspect of gay sex is that it is not confined by history. Heterosexual couples enter relationships having a basic understanding of what sex means to each of them and their roles. When two men have sex, the activities are more open-ended and can lead to any number of roles, positions, and actions. Because gay men have this sexual freedom, a whole kink subculture has evolved in the gay world that in-

*Gay*                                                           **33**

cludes a variety of sexual interests—leather, BDSM, puppy play, water sports, groups, and others.

Health professionals should be open-minded when talking about sex and sexuality with patients. Each patient will need to be assessed individually for what type of sex they have and who they have it with. Only then can a proper assessment be made about risk factors and health screenings. Be careful about the tone you are using when you ask questions; the way you ask a question can imply judgment: "You don't have bareback sex, do you?"

## BODY

Gay men and their bodies have a somewhat complicated relationship. In recent Western culture, gay men are held to the same standards as heterosexual women, in which physical appearance is generally considered to be of higher importance than personality, career, education, intelligence, and wealth. Many gay men try very hard to reach the ideal body image that Greek and Roman sculpture established long ago. Although this is not universal for all gay men, it exists enough as part of the gay culture to create body image concerns among many gay men. Gay men can develop body image issues that were previously thought to be isolated to women, and as a result, some gay men can develop eating disorders because of the social pressure to have a particular body type. In addition, plastic surgery and liposuction are becoming more mainstream for some gay men.

Many people might stereotypically envision gay men as superficial because of their focus on physical appearance, but although this focus can be a part of the culture, it certainly does not represent the gay population as a whole. In addition to this stereotyping, which might be to be considered negative, many gay men feel invisible because they do not fit into this category. Because they do not look and act a certain way, they think it means they are less gay or not gay at all. For young gay people, there is a need to fit in and find a community they belong to, which is complicated by the propagation of stereotypes.

There is a movement within the gay and queer community to be more accepting of all body types. Men of all sizes, races, and ethnic backgrounds are coming to understand that simply because they do not look like a classic sculpture, it does not mean they are unattractive to other gay men or, more importantly, unattractive to themselves. Communities are starting to move people away from the ideal of a "perfect body" and instead appreciate the diversity of bodies that exist.

## HIV

HIV, the human immunodeficiency virus, is intimately wrapped up in gay culture. This is true not because only gay people get the virus but because traditionally they are the most susceptible to it. Anal sex, in particular, is one of the more common ways the virus can be transmitted.

When HIV symptoms were first identified in the early 1980s, many people thought that the disease resulting from the virus was specific to gay men. This illness was initially termed gay-related immune deficiency (GRID). Gay men were dying by the thousands every year, and entire communities were wiped out by the disease. Many gay men lost their friends and lovers, leaving them isolated and alone in an already homophobic and rejecting world. After the virus was discovered, it took demonstrations and protests before money was dedicated to understanding the disease and how it is spread and to developing treatment options. Initial treatments such as AZT helped slow the transmission of HIV but had many side effects.

The culture around HIV became a significant part of the gay world from 1980 to the turn of the twenty-first century. In the past, before treatment for HIV was widely accessible, some men who wanted to let go of their fear or who wanted to be a part of a community would seek out opportunities to become HIV positive in the hopes of being connected with a part of the gay world. To date, more than 32 million people worldwide have died of HIV-related complications (World Health Organization 2019). The trauma caused by the death toll still has a lasting impact on the gay community, and emotional scars left on gay culture by the disease may never heal.

Times have changed, and our understanding of HIV has improved. Treatment options with fewer side effects are available, and people who are HIV positive are no longer dying in large numbers from complications of the disease. Although there is no cure, many people with HIV live life spans similar to those of individuals without HIV.

Despite treatment efforts, there remains a great deal of stigma in the gay community, and some gay men are terrified of contracting the disease. Many people who are HIV negative refer to themselves as "clean," implying that people who are HIV positive are dirty in some way. One way to combat stigma is through education. Many gay men have been educating themselves on what it means to be HIV positive, including information regarding viral load and CD4 count, and estimating risk on the basis of this information.

In recent years, PrEP has become more common as a means of preventing the spread of HIV. Individuals who are at risk of contracting HIV can now take antiretroviral medications, and many gay men who engage in sexual activity are opting to take PrEP as a way to protect themselves. Although PrEP is not 100% effective, it is very close to it, with rare cases of HIV transmission while someone is following the regimen. However, the emergence of PrEP has led to some problems. As a result of stigma attached to PrEP, some people believe that those taking PrEP are sexually promiscuous. In addition, some individuals think condom use is not necessary because they are taking PrEP, but several sexually transmitted diseases exist for which PrEP provides no protection. As a result of PrEP initiatives, HIV rates of transmission are dropping in large cities, but it is still unclear what will be the long-term implications of the intervention.

## SUBSTANCES

Substances and the gay community have a long history together. In many ways, commonly used substances such as alcohol have been intertwined into gay culture. As mentioned earlier in the chapter, gay men have limited ways of finding other gay men, especially in rural areas. Although there are more varied ways for gay men to meet today, traditionally a gay bar was one of the only safe spaces for gay people. As a result, alcohol was commonly available, and alcohol use was almost expected for many gay men.

Gay men have higher rates of substance abuse problems when compared with the general population (Ostrow and Stall 2008). However, some people believe the research on which these rates is based is flawed because finding gay-identified people in gay drinking establishments for research purposes does not give a realistic sample of all gay men (Bux 1996). The potential higher rates of substance abuse are largely thought to be related to minority stress (see the question "Are gay men more prone to mental illness and substance use" earlier in the chapter). Gay men in society are often labeled as "different" or "other" when compared with the larger heterosexual population. LGBTQ+ individuals have had to fight—and continue to fight—for their civil rights, such as job security and the ability to get married and have children, just to name a few. It is not difficult to understand why many would turn to alcohol and other drugs to escape their current situation or medicate symptoms with which they might be dealing.

Other drugs that are commercially available are becoming popular in gay culture. One example is poppers, an inhalant used by some gay men as a relaxant for their mind and body (see glossary earlier in the chapter). Many gay men say poppers help them relax for anal sex. Because these commercially available drugs are not regulated by the FDA, it is impossible to know what chemical compound is present. Overdose by inhaling poppers is rare, but they can be fatal if ingested.

Methamphetamine, or crystal meth, is another drug that has become associated with gay culture. Crystal meth can be seen as a "super cocaine," making the person who takes it feel energetic, euphoric, invincible, and very sexual. It is often paired with sexual encounters to enhance the positive feelings of sex. Although these effects might sound enticing to many people, crystal meth has significant health risks, including cardiac events, psychosis, and even death. Some gay men inject crystal meth, also called slamming, which can perpetuate these dangerous effects. Crystal meth use is also often linked to unprotected sexual encounters, increasing the spread of HIV and other sexually transmitted diseases.

It is necessary to talk to all patients about substances, but gay men should be given special attention considering their risk. Traditional Alcoholics Anonymous and other substance abuse programs might not be a welcoming place for a gay man, so treatment planning should consider the social aspects of care. When abstinence is not an option, harm reduction methods (e.g., condoms, PrEP) should be used whenever possible.

## CONVERSION THERAPY

Until the relatively recent past (see next subsection), homosexuality was seen as pathological and not a normal human variant. Previously, psychiatrists and other mental health care providers viewed a gay man's same-sex desire as something to fix or correct. The attempt to convert a person from being gay back to being straight is called *conversion therapy*.

Conversion is now known to be ineffective and dangerous. Sadly, some people who have gone through conversion therapy have taken their own lives. Changing a person's sexual orientation is not possible, and attempting to do so in a therapeutic setting is unethical. States are now passing laws that ban the practice of conversion therapy because of its known dangers.

Gay-affirming therapy is now the standard of care when working with gay men. A person's diverse sexual orientation should be viewed not as a pathology but as a unique part of the individual that should be expressed. Ultimately, the patient will identify their own sexual orientation, and the therapist's role is to help facilitate a safe space for them to identify their feelings and desires.

## HOMOSEXUALITY AND DSM

As mentioned in the previous subsection, homosexuality was thought to be a pathology and was listed as such in early printings of the second edition of the *Diagnostic and Statistical Manual of Mental Disorders* (DSM-II; American Psychiatric Association 1968). This controversial diagnosis remained in DSM until 1973, when it was removed after demonstrations and protests by gay activists (American Psychiatric Association 1973). It was also removed in part because of a speech that took place at the American Psychiatric Association (APA) in 1972. At the time, gay rights activists Barbara Gittings and Frank Kameny were working alongside gay-affirming psychiatrists to have homosexuality removed from DSM. At the 1972 APA annual meeting, Gittings and Kameny held a special symposium titled "Psychiatry: Friend or Foe of Homosexuals—A Dialogue." They were joined by a man wearing a mask, a fake wig, and a device to disguise his voice. He was referred to as Dr. H. Anonymous and spoke about his conflict with being both a psychiatrist and a homosexual. At the time, psychiatrists could lose their medical license for being homosexual because this was considered to be a mental disorder. Dr. H. Anonymous was John Fryer, M.D., a Philadelphia psychiatrist. His bravery, along with the work of Barbara Gittings and Frank Kameny, helped pave the way to depathologizing homosexuality.

## RELIGION AND SPIRITUALITY

Homosexuality and religion have had a long-complicated history. Although many religious communities are intolerant of homosexuality, it is important to avoid generalizing. Just as some religions may condemn or demonstrate hostility toward homosexuals, there are others that are accepting, or tolerant, of gay men, and still others that target specific acts (such as anal sex) without mention of sexuality. Even within a single religion, several factors may influence the varying degrees of tolerance demonstrated, such as the specific denomination or branch, interpretation and enforcement of religious scripture, and time period (as some religious subgroups become more progressive over time). Similarly, there are gay men in all religious affiliations, with varying degrees of religious involvement, and it is important to note that people may have different experiences even within similar communities. Regardless, exposure to religion, whether through family, community, or cultural environment, can deeply affect the identity development of a gay man.

With the prevalence of faiths conflating homosexuality and immorality, many gay men find themselves feeling conflicted about religion. These negative attitudes toward homosexuals create significant psychological distress, and this homophobia is often internalized, which may lead to restricted sexual and social development. Although some individuals may successfully reconcile or compartmentalize their spiritual and sexuality identities, others may switch to a more tolerant religion or abandon religion altogether. Others may continue to struggle with these conflicting identities into adulthood or may actively hinder their own sexual development to avoid religious estrangement. More recently, many gay men and allies have sought religious acceptance through activism, pushing religious reform or creating new religious or spiritual environments for LGBTQ+ members. This provides a welcoming environment otherwise often absent in more mainstream religious places and helps counter forced rejection and the guilt that comes with it.

## PARENTING

Gay men have always had children, whether from heterosexual relationships or in same-sex households. In the past 30 years, as politics have evolved and technology has advanced, gay men have been able to have children through several ways, including adoption, co-parenting, surrogacy, and donor insemination. Although the subject has been debated fervently, especially by politicians and religious leaders, studies have shown that gay men are as capable and fit as parents as heterosexual men (Crowl et al. 2008). Furthermore, empirical data show that children raised by gay men fare as well as those raised by heterosexual parents across several metrics, including physical and psychological health, cognitive development, and academic achievement.

Research also shows that being raised by same-sex couples does not influence the sexual orientation of children, and there are no differences in children's gender role behaviors compared with those of children raised in heterosexual families. As with children raised by straight couples, most children will grow up to self-identify as heterosexual. Some studies (e.g., Farr et al. 2017) do show that children raised by same-sex couples feel less pressured to follow traditional gender roles, and often they grow up in social environments that are more tolerant and less heterosexist. On the basis of the abundance of empirical evidence, many major international professional organizations (e.g., American Psychiatric Association, American Psychological Association, American Academy of Pediatrics) have issued statements in support of LGBTQ+ parental rights. However, despite this support, many gay men face significant inequity and legal discrimination, preventing them from becoming parents.

## RACE

Gay men are found among all races, ethnicities, and cultures, and this wide-sweeping diversity brings heterogeneity to gay culture. Racial and ethnic identity plays a significant role in an individual's development, experiences, and community belonging. In addition to belonging to a sexual minority, gay men of color have an added racial or ethnic minority identity in any white-dominated society. These distinct but interconnected identities are what is known as *double minority status*. Members of a double minority face unique stressors related to both identities individually as well as collectively, leading to internal and external conflicts.

Meyer (2003) described a stress model relevant to sexual minorities using a distal-proximal continuum. Distal stressors are objectively stressful events such as discrimination and harassment, including more subtle forms such as microaggressions, that affect the person externally. Proximal stressors involve subjective interpretation and internalization in relation to self-identity and negative societal attitudes. They may lead to negative self-respect, internalized shame, concealment of identity, and vigilance, with the expectation of rejection by others (Ramirez and Paz Galupo 2019).

The intersection of multiple stigmatized identities creates additional stressors targeting this multiple minority status, often leading to individuals feeling they do not belong or feeling forced to choose a primary identity. Individuals may confront or internalize homophobia and/or racism within their ethnic groups because some minority cultures may have prejudice toward other races/ethnicities and/or prevalent heterosexism. These dual minorities may also endure overt and covert racism within the gay community, which can take the form of white gays or other ethnic gays. Examples include discrimination through a proclaimed "preference" for whites only or fetishization for a specific ethnic group based on racist stereotypes. There is even homophobia within the larger gay community, often visible through forced heteronormativity and assumption of stereotypically male gender roles. The complexity of these conflicts can lead to intrapsychic and interpersonal detriment and may have a significant impact on successful identity development.

## AGING

With advances in medicine and public health come longer life expectancy and a pressing need for adequate geriatric care for the LGBT population. (Note that the Q is absent from the acronym here because some older LGBT adults were coming out when the word "queer" was being used primarily as a derogatory term. Only in the past decade has the term started to take on a positive connotation by representing a spectrum of sexual orientations and gender identities.) There are more than 3 million LGBT people older than age 55, and that number is increasing as the baby boomers age. Although the needs of an aging population change as priorities shift and individuals begin making long-term plans, special considerations are needed for aging LGBT adults. As people age, finding a community to be part of is important for individuals to find meaning and a sense of belonging. Isolation is a major issue among gay men, for a multitude of reasons. Before HIV diagnosis and treatment were as widely available, the illness ravaged the gay population because of the unknown mode of transmission. This led to the loss of countless lives and had devastating effects on victims, families, and friends.

Unfortunately, older gay men continue to face significant discrimination at assisted living and housing communities, often forcing them back into the closet. In addition, ageism within the gay community can further isolate LGBT elderly. Steps are being taken to tackle this problem as activists push for inclusion of sexual orientation protections and gay-friendly retirement communities pop up around the country. But there is still significant work to be done.

Because isolation is a significant risk factor for suicide, it is critical for clinicians to perform a thorough assessment of a patient's social structure, including risk of abuse and suicide. Older LGBT adults are more likely to be single and living alone than non-LGBT older adults. In addition to many living at or below the federal poverty line, older LGBT adults are more likely to be depressed, be substance users, and have major health problems. These components may provide a clinician significant information about a patient's health, both physically and mentally, so that concerns may be addressed early on.

## FAMILY OF CHOICE

Many gay men come from parts of the country and the world that are not accepting of diverse sexual orientations. Even within supportive environments, biological families might not be accepting of their gay family member because of cultural or religious reasons. Because of his, many gay people find a *family of choice*—a group of individuals who provide support, largely emotional support. When working with patients who are gay men, clinicians should be mindful of who might be the patient's most supportive family members. Sometimes, gay patients want the clinician to be in contact with their family of choice rather than their biological family because the biological family may increase stress and symptoms.

# Conclusion

The culture around gay men has a complicated past, with most of its history treating them with hate and prejudice. As gay men feel safer to come out, their culture and people's reaction to it has grown in positive and negative ways. Gay men face external opinions and beliefs about their own identities—before they can form them themselves—sometimes contributing to internalized homophobia.

# FIVE TAKE-HOME POINTS

- The word *gay* is very broad and can refer to someone's sexual behavior, sexual identity, and/or social constructs or an entire subculture.

- Gay men have experienced persecution and discrimination throughout history, which still continues in the United States and most parts of the world.

- Internalized homophobia is the internalization of negative societal opinions about gay people and can occur within LGBTQ+ individuals as well as straight people.

- Gay patients will have their own beliefs and values; clinicians should be careful not to project their own values onto patients.

- Gay men are multilayered, and the gay community experiences complications within many aspects of personhood, including religion, race, sex, drug use, and age.

## Resources

It Gets Better Project, https://itgetsbetter.org
Lambda Legal, https://lambdalegal.org
LGBT National Help Center, http://glbtnationalhelpcenter.org
National LGBT Health Education Center, https://lgbthealth
    education.org
The Trevor Project, https://thetrevorproject.org

## References

American Psychiatric Association: Diagnostic and Statistical Manual of Mental Disorders, 2nd Edition. Washington, DC, American Psychiatric Association, 1968

American Psychiatric Association: Homosexuality and sexual orientation disturbance: proposed change in DSM-II, 6th printing, page 44. APA Document Ref No 730008. Washington, DC, American Psychiatric Association, 1973. Available at: https://dsm.psychiatry online.org/doi/pdf/10.1176/appi.books.9780890420362.dsm-ii-6thprintingchange. Accessed: November 25, 2019.

Bux DA Jr: The epidemiology of problem drinking in gay men and lesbians: a critical review. Clin Psychol Rev 16(4):277–298, 1996

Crowl A, Ahn S, Baker J: A meta-analysis of developmental outcomes for children of same-sex and heterosexual parents. J GLBT Fam Stud 4:(3)385–407, 2008

Drescher J: Psychoanalytic Therapy and the Gay Man. Mahwah, NJ, Analytic Press, 2001

Eckstrand KL, Ehrenfeld JM (eds): Lesbian, Gay, Bisexual, and Transgender Healthcare: A Clinical Guide to Preventive, Primary, and Specialist Care. New York, Springer, 2016

Farr RH, Bruun ST, Doss KM, Patterson CJ: Children's gender-typed behavior from early to middle childhood in adoptive families with lesbian, gay, and heterosexual parents. Sex Roles 78(7–8):528–541, 2017

Hamel L, Firth J, Hoff T, et al: HIV/AIDS in the Lives of Gay and Bisexual Men in the United States. Menlo Park, CA, Henry J. Kaiser Family Foundation, September 2014. Available at: http://files.kff.org/attachment/survey-hivaids-in-the-lives-of-gay-and-bisexual-men-in-the-united-states. Accessed January 30, 2020.

Horowitz JL, Newcomb MD: A multidimensional approach to homosexual identity. J Homosex 42(2):1–19, 2002

Joyner K, Manning WD, Bogle RH: Gender and the stability of same-sex and different-sex relationships among young adults. Demography 54(6)2351–2374, 2017

Levounis P, Drescher J, Barber ME (eds): The LGBT Casebook. Washington, DC, American Psychiatric Publishing, 2012

Meyer IH: Prejudice, social stress, and mental health in lesbian, gay, and bisexual populations: conceptual issues and research evidence. Psychol Bull 129(5):674–697, 2003

Mustanski BS, Garofalo R, Emerson EM: Mental health disorders, psychological distress, and suicidality in a diverse sample of lesbian, gay, bisexual, and transgender youths. Am J Public Health 100(12):2426–2432, 2010 20966378

NPR, Robert Woods Johnson Foundation, Harvard TH Chan School of Public Health: Discrimination in America: Experiences and Views of LGBTQ Americans. November 2017. Available at: www.npr.org/documents/2017/nov/npr-discrimination-lgbtq-final.pdf. Accessed January 30, 2020.

Ostrow DG, Stall R: Alcohol, tobacco, and drug use among gay and bisexual men, in Unequal Opportunity: Health Disparities Affecting Gay and Bisexual Men in the United States. Edited by Wolitski RJ, Stall R, Valdiserri RO. New York, Oxford University Press, 2008

Ramirez JL, Paz Galupo M: Multiple minority stress: the role of proximal and distal stress on mental health outcomes among lesbian, gay, and bisexual people of color. J Gay Lesbian Ment Health 23(2):145–167, 2019

Rosario M, Schrimshaw EW, Hunter J, Braun L: Sexual identity development among gay, lesbian, and bisexual youths: consistency and change over time. J Sex Res 43(1):46–58, 2006

World Health Organization: HIV/AIDS fact sheet. Geneva, Switzerland, World Health Organization, November 15, 2019. Available at: www.who.int/news-room/fact-sheets/detail/hiv-aids. Accessed February 25, 2020.

# Chapter 3

# Bisexual

## *The B in LGBTQ²IAPA*

SARAH NOBLE, D.O.

Freud's most radical legacy is the one that is the least actualized. After years of evolution on the topic, he came to the conclusion that any exclusive monosexual interest—-regardless of whether it was hetero- or homosexual—was neurotic. In a sense Freud is saying what second-wave critic Kate Millet said a half-century late: "Homosexuality was invented by a straight world dealing with its own bisexuality." By the end of his writings, in 1937, Freud was downright blithe about bisexuality: "Every human being['s]...libido is distributed, either in a manifest or a latent fashion, over objects of both sexes."

*Jennifer Baumgardner, Look Both Ways: Bisexual Politics*

There are not two discreet populations, heterosexual and homosexual...only the human mind invents categories and tries to force fact into separated pigeon holes... The sooner we learn this concerning sexual behavior, the sooner we shall reach a sound understanding of the realities of sex.

*Alfred Kinsey, Sexual Behavior in the Human Male, 1948*

## Psychological and Cultural Context

As an introduction to this chapter on bisexuality, let us first review some of the most pervasive myths about bisexuals.

These beliefs can be found not only in heteronormative culture but in the gay world as well.

- Bisexuality is just a phase (e.g., a lesbian until graduation or gay but in the closet)
- Bisexuals cannot be faithful
- Only women are bisexual, not men
- A person cannot identify as bisexual unless they have had a sexual relationship with both a man and a woman
- Bisexuals are not as oppressed as gay men or lesbians because they have straight privilege

We will discuss why these statements are untrue later in the chapter, but first, in order to understand why these myths are so pervasive, we must look at the history of sexuality in Western society.

Bisexual behavior has existed in recorded culture since both ancient Greek and Roman times as well as in ancient Japan. It is well known that both Greek and Roman men married women but took young men for lovers. In Japan, same-sex relationships between older and younger men were also an accepted practice during the Edo period (1603–1867). These relationships, called nanshoku, were represented in writing by a character that means sexual pleasure. Far from being stigmatized or understood as deviant, lust or bodily desire of all kinds was believed to be common to all men. As David Halperin says of ancient Greece and Rome, "a male desire to pursue sexual contact with other males without impugning in the slightest his own masculinity or normative identity as a man…" was common (Halperin 1998).

Throughout modern history in Europe, however, a series of laws and religious canon expressly forbade sexually "deviant" acts such as sodomy. Foucault writes of this in his History of Sexuality, stating, "up to the end of the eighteenth century, three major explicit codes—apart from the regularity of custom and constraints of opinion—governed sexual practices: canon law, Christian pastoral, and civil law" (Halperin 1998, p. 98).

In the late 1800s, scientists first began to use the term *bisexual*, but in a very different sense from our usage today. The word referred to an organism's ability to develop into the male or female of the species. When it was discovered that humans do not differentiate into male or female until the 12th week of gestation, the term was applied to humans as well

(Rapoport 2009). Thus, the original use of the term was actually a reference to sex and not to sexual orientation. When Freud began to use the term, he appeared to extend the physical into the psychological realm so that "bisexuality implied both bigenderism and dual attraction" (Rapoport 2009, p. 282).

For Freud, the child begins, as does the embryo, with the potential for feminine and masculine identity, but the child must mature through identification with the appropriate parent and become a healthy adult. Freud's theory of immaturity designates both homosexuals and bisexuals as fixated or regressed. "Nevertheless, his approach had a somewhat inclusive quality—the homosexual within is a necessary part of heterosexual development" (Drescher 2004). Steven Angelides, author of *A History of Bisexuality*, argues, however, that "Freud's placement of bisexuality in the past (of the individual and the species) [is] an example of a pervasive cultural phenomenon that he called 'erasure of bisexuality in the present tense'" (Rapoport 2009, p. 282). In other words, although all humans begin with this potential for bisexuality, it is only healthy heterosexuals who go on to sublimate their attraction to the same sex so that they can reproduce and perpetuate the species.

By relegating bisexuality (as well as homosexuality) to the neurotic and hysteric patient, Freud created the groundwork for yet a fourth code to govern sexual practice.

> The nineteenth-century prohibitions against homosexuality, which did not simply criminalize sexual relations between men as illegal, but medically disqualified them as pathological and—not content with penalizing the act—constructed the perpetrator as a deviant form of life, a perverse personality, an anomalous species, thereby producing a new specification of individuals whose true nature would be defined from now on by referencing their abnormal sexuality. (Halperin 1998, p. 98)

Freud himself, however, seemed loath to actually condemn homosexuality, famously saying to a mother who wrote to him about her gay son,

> homosexuality is assuredly no advantage, but it is nothing to be ashamed of, no vice, no degradation; it cannot be classified as an illness; we consider it to be a variation of the sexual function, produced by a certain arrest of sexual development. Many highly respectable individuals of ancient and modern times have been homosexuals, several of the greatest men

*Bisexual*

among them (Plato, Michelangelo, Leonardo da Vinci, etc.).
It is a great injustice to persecute homosexuality as a crime—
and a cruelty, too" (Freud 1935)

However, 10 years later, the field of psychoanalysis deemed Freud's model of the bisexual or hermaphrodite embryo to be flawed and moved fully toward pathologizing homosexuality (Hire et al. 2012).

Thus, we see that although bisexuality was generally accepted in ancient Rome and Greece, where "amorous behavior was considered an art whose forms and styles of expression were infinite" (Alexander and Anderlini-D'Onofrio 2009), it came to be vilified in Western culture through a number of hegemonies. As "Nature came to be studied scientifically in modernity under the aegis of Christian monotheism" (Alexander and Anderlini-D'Onofrio 2009, p. 463), both religious and civil laws regarding sexual behavior were created to curtail sexuality. With the advent of Freud's theories of sexuality, yet another method of limitation had been created: that of the scientific and medical heuristic within which deviation is equated with illness and pathology.

It was not until the 1940s and 1950s that Albert Kinsey's important research on bisexuality challenged the notion that it was only a few pathological people who continued to be bisexual into adulthood because of neurosis or hysteria. In his research on 11,000 people, Kinsey found that "28% of women and 46% of men had responded erotically or were sexually active with both women and men" (Beemyn 2004). Kinsey also developed a scale to illustrate the degree to which someone was attracted to one gender or the other.

Throughout the 1960s, 1970s, and 1980s, as the gay civil rights movement was growing in the United States, the bisexual rights movement matured alongside it. However, bisexuality remained problematic even for the gay and lesbian rights community: "…[T]he in-between status of bisexuality seems to question too much the nonthreatening innateness upon which much of gay politicking came to depend. We're born this way, after all, so please don't discriminate" (Alexander and Anderlini-D'Onofrio 2009, p. 464). Yet as Lisa Diamond says, "how, why, when, and for how long someone is LGBT may be fascinating to a scientist like me, but it should have no bearing on public policy. We all deserve acceptance and equality" (Diamond 2018).

# Questions Well-Meaning People Ask

### Is bisexuality just a phase?

This question has its origins in Freud's ideas about psychosexuality and the psychoanalytic schools on which the field of psychiatry is based. Rather than accepting that, as Kinsey's research has shown, people have a diverse range of sexual attractions, the Freudian notion that heterosexuality is the mature state toward which bisexuals need to be guided with therapy has infiltrated the collective unconscious. This myth is then used by straight and gay people alike to erase bisexual identity, or to create *bi-erasure*. In fact, research by Lisa Diamond of a group of women who identified as lesbian, bisexual, or unlabeled over a 10-year period showed that "bisexuality can best be interpreted as a stable pattern of attraction to both sexes in which the specific balance of same-sex and other-sex desires necessarily varies according to interpersonal and situational factors" (Diamond 2008).

### Can bisexuals be faithful?

Yes. This question may reflect *biphobia*, which is an aversion toward bisexuality and bisexual people as a social group or as individuals. It can take the form of denial that bisexuality is a genuine sexual orientation or of negative stereotypes about people who are bisexual (such as beliefs that they are promiscuous or dishonest).

Marjorie Garber spoke eloquently to this issue in her text Vice Versa: "those who confuse or conflate bisexuality with non-monogamy or non-monogamy with group sex, tend to think of it as a tangle of bodies or body parts. This is not only because the fantasy of three-in-a-bed is exciting… but also because of the difficulty of visualizing or conceptualizing bisexuality except as triadic, triangular, kinetic, or peripatetic" (Garber 1995). The idea that bisexuals cannot be faithful becomes a vehicle for biphobia. Again, in her longitudinal study of women's attractions, Diamond (2008) found that "not only did bisexual women tend to pursue exclusive, monogamous relationships over time, but they were more likely to do so than either unlabeled or lesbian women" (p. 13).

### Is it true that only women are bisexual, not men?

No. A 2016 Centers for Disease Control and Prevention National Health Statistics Report stated that 2% of American men ages

18–44 years reported being bisexual (95.1% reported being straight, and 1.9% reported being gay) (Copen et al. 2016). Given the population of the United States, this means that there are more than 3 million bisexual men, almost equivalent to the population of Idaho. It is also likely that social factors affect the visibility of bisexual men. "The past decade has witnessed a notable increase in television and film portrayals of heterosexually identified women engaging in experimental same-sex behavior, usually with few negative consequences" (Diamond 2012), but we do not see a corresponding acceptance of same-sex sexual behavior among men in pop culture. We cannot conclusively state that the data mean there are more bisexual women than men because the data could be the consequence of years of depictions of women as pop culture sex objects as well as a culture of toxic masculinity, with its assumption that men must be other-sex attracted.

**Can someone identify as bisexual if they have not had a relationship with both a man and a woman?**

Yes. The problem with this question is that it conflates the fairly straightforward *relationship status* with the much more complex notion of *identity*, a multifaceted conception of oneself that can include gender and sexual orientation as well as race, ethnicity, profession, parenthood, and many other things. The conflation of lived experience with identity, the assumption that bisexuality requires a relationship history with both men and women, may not take into account other events or limitations that might have occurred in an individual's life. For instance, a man who identifies as bisexual might have met a woman at age 18, started a monogamous relationship with her, and chose not to date anyone since. This doesn't negate his bisexuality, but it may simply reflect the lack of opportunity to explore those desires. Likewise, a woman who identifies as bisexual may live in a small community and have very few opportunities to explore relationships with other LGBTQ+ people, and thus has been limited to heterosexual relationships throughout her life. Again, identity does not change despite the situational limitations of someone's environment and history.

**Is it true that bisexuals aren't as oppressed as gays or lesbians because they have straight privilege?**

No. In fact, among the lesbian, gay, and bisexual (LGB) family, bisexuals often have the worst health outcomes. Bisexual women similarly report worse mental health and suicidality than lesbians and heterosexual women (Kerr et al. 2013). In comparison with heterosexual and lesbian women, bisexual women are more likely to report feeling overwhelming anxiety, exhaustion, and hopelessness. Compared with heterosexual males, bisexual males have 143%–204% the odds of being threatened or injured with a weapon (Friedman et al. 2011). They are also 24%–57% more likely than exclusively homosexual males to suffer these forms of bullying . These differences occur because bisexuals can feel doubly excluded: not only do they have to tolerate homophobia, but they also experience bi-erasure and biphobia from the lesbian and gay community. As we know from the minority stress model (see Chapter 2, "Gay"), the more levels of minority status held by an individual, the more likely they are to have struggles with mental health problems (Meyer 2003).

## Themes That May Emerge in Therapy

It is quite likely that in your practice you will work with patients who are either bisexual or attracted to the same sex. As we can see from the 2016 Centers for Disease Control and Prevention (CDC) data, although only 5.5% of women and 2% of men identify as bisexual, a significantly larger portion of the population acknowledge same-sex behavior (17.4% for women and 6.2% for men) (Copen et al. 2016).

When treating any patient, it is important to remember that not only do we have to challenge ourselves to overcome the common myths around bisexuality, but our patients might need to overcome these myths as well. We theorize that one of the reasons there is such a large disparity between the number of people who identify as bisexual and those who express same-sex behavior is internalized biphobia. As therapists, we may need to help patients work through shame, negative attitudes, or internalized myths to actualize their identity. This might involve coming out to family members or a spouse or just acknowledging to themselves their sexual orientation.

### COMING OUT

Coming out is a well-theorized process and typically involves recognizing same-sex attraction and then finding a community of other lesbians and gays, becoming immersed in that community, and then finally integrating one's sexual orientation into one's identity. Bisexuals experience a number of these phases, but the process can often be complicated by biphobia or bi-erasure within the lesbian and gay community. In addition, attraction to opposite-sex partners can be interpreted in different and conflicted ways for many bisexuals. Thus, the path to identity formation that traditionally happens during adolescence can often take varied paths for people with bisexual attraction. A MetLife study of baby boomers indicates that by their later life, only 16% of bisexuals are completely out compared with close to 80% of lesbians and gays (MetLife Mature Market Institute 2010).

## RACE AND INTERSECTIONALITY

One of the most well-known communities of closeted bisexuals is *down low* men. These are African American men who identify as heterosexual but have sex with men. Often, they identify pressures such as cultural norms or religious values as the reasons for not coming out as bisexual. Although down low men are traditionally identified as vectors for HIV/AIDS transmission, a recent CDC study indicates that this population is no more likely than their heterosexual counterparts to spread HIV (Bond et al. 2009).

As mentioned previously, the minority stress model indicates that the more levels of minority status an individual has, the more risk factors that person has for mental health problems. The model also takes into account protective factors such as community supports from members of the same minority group. Thus, we can see the instinctive protective drive for African American men to protect themselves from a dual minority status by staying on the down low.

## SUBSTANCE USE

Bisexuals have increased risk of substance use, likely due to increased minority status, bi-erasure, and biphobia. One study found prevalence of problem-drinking patterns to be 31.2% and of illicit substance use to be 30.5% (Ross et al. 2014). Therefore, when treating people who identify as bisexual, it important to screen for substance use as a method for coping with minority stress.

## SEXUALITY AND RELATIONSHIPS

Possibly because of aforementioned ideas such as conflating bisexuality with non-monogamy and polyamory, we often associate bisexuals with hypersexuality. However, it is likely that at least a percentage of bisexuals are also asexual. Unfortunately, because of a dearth of research on asexuality, we do not have good data on the cross-over. Poston and Baumle (2010) did an exhaustive analysis of data from the 2002 National Survey of Family Growth to try to determine the prevalence of asexuality in the United States and found that 5% of women and 6% of men have never had sex in their lifetime. It is reasonable to assume that some of these people identify as bisexual, although we do not have data on the percentage.

Some bisexual patients will be involved in polyamory or open relationships. Polyamory differs from non-monogamy, which is an umbrella term for any nondyadic relationship. Non-monogamy can include swinging, cheating, or consensual open relationships such as polyamory. Polyamory is based on the idea that a person can meet all of the relationship needs of more than one person. Because of stigma around cultural norms, these people are often hesitant to talk about their relationships. Treating therapists are often biased toward monogamy, and "because of this bias, they are often tempted to focus on changing the lifestyle rather than on alleviating the specific problems that motivated the individual to seek counseling to begin with" (Johnson 2013).

## PARENTING AND FAMILIES

Parenting is often very difficult for bisexuals because although our world has adapted to the idea of same-sex couples, bisexual couples are still not a common concept. However, data indicate that more bisexual people are parenting than lesbians and gays. Fifty-nine percent of bisexual women and 32% of bisexual men have had kids, compared to 31% of lesbians and 16% of gay men (Goldberg et al. 2014). Because bisexual people make up the largest portion of the LGB community, this means that more than two-thirds of LGB parents are bisexual. Often, bisexuals find they are parenting with opposite-sex partners because the reality is that the majority of the dating pool is straight. This contributes to the sense that bisexuality is a phase and to the occurrence of bi-erasure during this important developmental life phase.

As therapists, it is our role to guide our patients through the task of maintaining or shifting identities as needed, as well as searching for community supports. As therapists, our role is to guide patients through the task of maintaining or shifting identities as needed. We can also create a holding environment as patients search for solid community supports.

AGING

As with all communities with whom we work, aging brings with it issues of loss, regret, and grief as well as consolidation of identity. Older bisexual adults show shocking levels of poverty rates matched only by older transgender adults. Forty-seven percent of bisexuals older than 65 years and 48% of trans people older than 65 years live at or below 200% of the poverty level. By comparison, only about 33% of age-matched lesbians and gays live at or below 200% of the poverty level (Movement Advancement Project 2017). A MetLife study looking at baby boomers and their family of choice found that although lesbian and gay boomers had an average of six close friends, bisexuals had only four (MetLife Mature Market Institute 2010). When looking at who had needed care from a friend or family member in the last 6 months because of a health problem or condition, gay men were about half as likely to have recently needed care (9%) compared with bisexual men and women (17%) and lesbians and transgender people (19%).

# Conclusion

The human brain is most comfortable working in binaries: male/female, heterosexual/homosexual. Bisexuality, by its very nature, is an identity that challenges simple categorization. Not only do people experience attraction to more than one gender, but their degree of attraction might vary, and it might shift throughout their life. This slipperiness causes discomfort for even the most open-minded among us. As Garber says, bisexuality "encompasses too much; it does not try to resolve contradictions but to accept them. It tells, we might say, too many stories, when what is so ardently desired, [is] the real story" (Garber 1995). Perhaps, she suggests, "bisexuality is a third kind of sexual identity, or beyond homosexuality and heterosexuality?… Why instead of hetero-, homo-, auto-, pan-, and bisexuality, do we not simply say 'sexuality?'" (Garber 1995). In other words, why not for once and for all let go of the insistence on categorization and move forward by accepting that bodies are sexual?

As Diamond (2016) has shown in her work,

> between 25 and 75% of individuals reported substantial changes in their attractions over time, and these findings concord with the results of retrospective studies showing that gay, lesbian, and bisexual-identified individuals commonly recall having undergone previous shifts in their attractions. Such findings pose a powerful corrective to previous oversimplification of sexual orientation as a fundamentally stable and rigidly categorical phenomenon. (p. 250)

In other words, sexual orientation does not rigidly predict each and every desire an individual will experience over a lifespan; rather, "sexual fluidity represents a context-dependent capacity for change in attraction" (Diamond 2016, p. 250).

Perhaps recognizing this fluidity would give us the space to work with our patients on their emotional connections and supports, as well as their personal identities and role development. After all, when it comes down to it, bisexual patients still must go through all the major life stages that any other person does. They must separate and individuate, find their professional and romantic identities, decide whether they want to start families, and then create lasting and satisfying identities through old age. Our job as therapists is to help them do this among and despite the biphobia and bi-erasure that currently exist in our culture.

# FIVE TAKE-HOME POINTS

- Bisexuality is not a phase.
- Bisexuals suffer from biphobia and bi-erasure from both the straight world and from lesbians and gays.
- Because of the stigma of bisexuality, most bisexuals do not come out.
- Bisexuals suffer from substance use disorders and other mental health disorders at higher rates than do their heterosexual and homosexual peers
- Sexual orientation may change over a person's lifespan.

# Resources

## U.S. NATIONAL ORGANIZATIONS

BiNet USA, www.binetusa.org
Bisexual.org, https://bisexual.org
Bisexual Resource Center, https://biresource.org

## EDUCATIONAL RESOURCES

Bi Magazine, https://bisexual.org/blog
Bisexual Organizing Project, www.bisexualorganizing
    project.org
*Journal of Bisexuality*, www.tandfonline.com/toc/wjbi20/
    .UaDtKOse5Xk

# References

Alexander J, Anderlini-D'Onofrio A: We are everywhere: a five-way review of A History of Bisexuality, Open, Becoming Visible, Bisexual Spaces, and Look Both Ways. J Bisex 9(3–4):461–476, 2009

Beemyn BG: Bisexuality. 2004. Available at www.glbtqarchive.com/ssh/bisex_S.pdf. Accessed February 2, 2020.

Bond L, Wheeler DP, Millett GA, et al: Black men who have sex with men and the association of down-low identity with HIV risk behavior. Am J Public Health 99(suppl 1):S92–S95, 2009

Copen CE, Chandra A, Febo-Vazquez I: Sexual behavior, sexual attraction, and sexual orientation among adults aged 18–44 in the United States: data from the 2011–2013 National Survey of Family Growth. Natl Health Stat Rep Jan 7(88):1–14, 2016 26766410

Diamond LM: Female bisexuality from adolescence to adulthood: results from a 10-year longitudinal study. Dev Psychol 44(1):5–14, 2008

Diamond LM: The desire disorder in research on sexual orientation in women: contributions of dynamical systems theory. Arch Sex Behav 41(1):73–83, 2012

Diamond LM: Sexual fluidity in males and females. Curr Sex Health Rep 8(4):249–256, 2016

Diamond L: Why the "born this way" argument doesn't advance LGBT equality (video). TEDxSaltLakeCity, December 18, 2018. Available at: www.youtube.com/watch?v=RjX-KBPmgg4. Accessed February 2, 2020.

Drescher J: Homosexuality and its vicissitudes: the "homosexual other" in psychoanalytic theory and praxis. Paper presented at Embodied Psyches/Life Politics Seminar Series, Centre for the Study of Invention and Social Process, Goldsmiths College, University of London, London, October 15, 2004

Freud S: Sigmund Freud writes to concerned mother: "Homosexuality is nothing to be ashamed of." (1935), Open Culture, September 26, 2014. Available at: www.openculture.com/2014/09/freud-letter-on-homosexuality.html. Accessed February 2, 2020.

Friedman MS, Marshal MP, Guadamuz TE, et al: A meta-analysis of disparities in childhood sexual abuse, parental physical abuse, and peer victimization among sexual minority and sexual nonminority individuals. Am J Public Health 101(8):1481–1494, 2011

Garber M: From Vice Versa: Bisexuality and the Eroticism of Everyday Life, 1995. Available at: https://prelectur.stanford.edu/lecturers/garber/viceversa.html. Accessed February 2, 2020.

Goldberg AE, Gartrell NK, Gates G: Research report on LGB-parent families. Los Angeles, CA, Williams Institute, UCLA School of Law, July 2014. Available at: http://williamsinstitute.law.ucla.edu/wp-content/uploads/lgb-parent-families-july 2014.pdf. Accessed February 2, 2020.

Halperin DM: Forgetting Foucault: acts, identities, and the history of sexuality. Representations 63(summer):93–120, 1998

Hire R, Rosario VA, Barber M, et al: The History of Psychiatry and Homosexuality. LGBT Mental Health Syllabus. Dallas, TX, Group for the Advancement of Psychiatry, 2012. Available at: http://www.aglp.org/gap/1_history/. Accessed February 2, 2020.

Johnson AL: Counseling the polyamorous client: implications for competent practice. Vistas Online, Article 50, Alexandria, VA, American Counseling Association, 2013. Available at www.counseling.org/docs/default-source/vistas/counseling-the-polyamorous-client-implications.pdf?sfvrsn=9. Accessed February 2, 2020.

Kerr DL, Santurri L, Peters P: Comparison of lesbian, bisexual, and heterosexual college undergraduate women on selected mental health issues. J Am Coll Health 61(4):185–194, 2013

MetLife Mature Market Institute: Still Out, Still Aging: The MetLife Study of Lesbian, Gay, Bisexual, and Transgender Baby Boomers. New York, MetLife Mature Market Institute, March 2010. Available at: www.giaging.org/documents/mmi-still-out-still-aging.pdf. Accessed February 2, 2020.

Meyer IH: Prejudice, social stress, and mental health in lesbian, gay, and bisexual populations: conceptual issues and research evidence. Psychol Bull 129(5):674–697, 2003

Movement Advancement Project, BiNetUSA, Bisexual Organizing Project, Bisexual Resource Center, SAGE: A closer look: bisexual older adults. Boulder, CO, Movement Advancement Project, September 2017. Available at: www.lgbtmap.org/file/A%20Closer%20Look%20Bisexual%20Older%20Adults%20FINAL.pdf. Accessed February 2, 2020.

Poston DL, Baumle A: Patterns of asexuality in the United States. Demographic Research 23(18):509–553, 2010

Rapoport E: Bisexuality in psychoanalytic therapy: interpreting the resistance. J Bisex 9(3–4):279–295, 2009

*Bisexual*

Ross LF, Bauer GR, MacLeod MA, et al: Mental health and substance use among bisexual youth and non-youth in Ontario, Canada. PLoS One 9(8):e101604, 2014

# Chapter 4

# Transgender

## The T in LGBTQ²IAPA

MURAT ALTINAY, M.D.

So you got two choices: Do the con, like I said,
or you gotta bite the big one. Either you do the boy thing or
you gotta snuff yourself. That's the way the world works,
my friend, and you ain't about to change it.

*Christine Howey,* Exact Change *(2017 film)*

## Psychological and Cultural Context

### TERMINOLOGY

The term *transgender* traditionally has been used when an individual's assigned gender at birth does not match the gender they experience themself to be. The term can be broader, however, referring to people of various gender identities. In contrast, the term *cisgender* refers to individuals who identify with their biological sex or the sex assigned at birth. In order to have a better understanding of the transgender community, it is important to clarify some basic concepts and definitions, such as chromosomal sex, biological sex, gender identity, gender expression, and sexual orientation (Table 4–1). Although Table 4–1 provides a general guideline for understanding gender and nonbinary representations, it is best to always approach people as individuals and understand that everyone has unique ways of expressing and identifying themselves.

**TABLE 4–1.** Common LGBTQ+ terminology

| Term | Definition |
| --- | --- |
| **Sex** | |
| Chromosomal sex | Karyotype (i.e., 46 XX, 46 XY, and all of the other variations) of an individual |
| Biological sex | Determined by the genitalia individuals are born with<br>• Includes internal and external genitalia<br>• Internal and external genitalia can develop separately<br>• Genitalia can be described as male, female, or ambiguous<br>• Individuals with ambiguous genitalia are also referred to as intersex |
| **Gender identity** | |
| Cisgender | Individuals who identify with their assigned gender at birth, which matches their biological and chromosomal sex |
| Transgender binary | Individuals who identify with the opposite end of their biological/assigned gender at birth, which does not match their biological and chromosomal sex (i.e., transgender male, transgender female) |
| Transgender nonbinary | Individuals who identify with a gender that does not fall in one of the polar ends of the gender spectrum, including the following identities:<br>• Agender<br>• Nongender<br>• Genderqueer<br>• Androgynous<br>• Feminine male<br>• Masculine female<br>• Transmasculine<br>• Transfeminine |

*Gender identity* is conceptualized as how masculine or how feminine a person is. A person can be both masculine and feminine or neither as well. *Gender expression* refers to the tools an individual uses to express their gender to the outside world regardless of the biological and chromosomal sex and gender identity (e.g., an individual is born male, identifies as female, and has gender-neutral [androgynous] expression). *Sexual orientation* describes whom an individual is attracted to sexually or emotionally. Some of the common terms (among many others) used to describe sexual orientation include heterosexual (attracted to opposite sex), homosexual (attracted to same sex), bisexual (equally attracted to both male and female sex), asexual (not attracted to any sex), and pansexual (attracted to all binary and nonbinary sexes). Given the complexity of gender identity and expression, more open terms such as *attracted to maleness/masculinity* or *attracted to femaleness/femininity* are also used and can be a more inclusive way to describe sexual orientation.

Transgender people experience incongruence between their assigned gender at birth and their identified gender and use a wide variety of terminology to express their gender identity. These terms could broadly be divided into two categories: *binary* and *nonbinary* gender identity. Binary gender terms include the two polar ends of the gender spectrum: male and female. Transgender people who identify themselves as binary use terms such as *male* (or *trans male*) or *female* (or *trans female*) to describe their gender identity, whereas people who do not experience gender in binary terms use a wide range of terminology to identify their gender identity (*agender, nongender, genderqueer, androgynous, feminine male, masculine female, transmasculine, transfeminine,* and many others). For binary transgender people who have not started the gender transition (gender affirmation) process or for people in the process of transitioning, the terms *male to female* (MTF) and *female to male* (FTM) are frequently used to specify the biological gender and the experienced (identified/end goal) gender. For nonbinary people, the term nonbinary is used, followed by the individual's specific gender identity description (e.g., nonbinary transmasculine). It is worthwhile noting that gender identity can fluctuate and change over time. Therefore, rather than thinking of these concepts as rigid, static notions, seeing them as ever-evolving, ever-changing concepts leads to a better understanding of transgender individuals, avoidance of mistakes and assumptions, and better patient care.

In addition to their gender identity, transgender people also vary in sexual orientation (homosexual, heterosexual, pansexual, asexual) and gender expression (feminine, masculine, androgynous). It is worth mentioning that, similar to gender identity, sexual orientation is also not a static, rigid concept and changes over time. This dynamic concept was first introduced by American researcher Fritz Klein (Klein et al. 1985), who criticized the static nature of the Kinsey scale (Kinsey et al. 2003) and added *past, present,* and *idealized future* items on his scale, acknowledging the concept that sexual orientation can change over time. For clinicians to understand the transgender population as a whole, understanding sexual orientation and its dynamic nature in this population is extremely important. Given the complexity and variety of identification possibilities, clarification of all of these terms not only leads to a healthier relationship with transgender individuals but also helps identify and reduce risk factors. In addition, because gender expression is a dynamic concept, it may or may not be a direct representation of an individual's current gender identity, sexual orientation, mood, and social environment.

Another important concept to mention is *gender pronouns* (Table 4–2). Gender pronouns are divided into three broad categories: 1) female pronouns (she/her/hers), 2) male pronouns (he/him/his), and 3) nonbinary pronouns (e.g., singular they/them/their, one, ze, sie, hir). Considering the fluidity of gender identity and gender expression, transgender individuals may or may not use pronouns that match their biological, experienced, or expressed gender (e.g., a biological female may identify as male, appear feminine, and use nonbinary pronouns); it is therefore important for clinicians to ask individuals about their pronouns in order to avoid mistakes.

## GENDER DYSPHORIA

Transgender people experience incongruence between their biological (assigned) gender and experienced (identified) gender (Meyer-Bahlburg 2010). When the incongruence between the experienced gender and the gender assigned at birth causes significant impairment in psychological, social,

**TABLE 4–2.** Gender pronouns

|  | Subject | Object | Possessive |
|---|---|---|---|
| Gender binary | She | Her | Hers |
|  | He | Him | His |
| Gender neutral | They | Them | Their |
|  | Ze | Hir | Hir |
|  | Xe | Xem | Xyr |
|  | Ze | Zir | Zir |

and occupational functioning, the term *gender dysphoria* is used. Previously, this condition was known as gender identity disorder. This term led to misperceptions, giving some people the impression that there might be an underlying characterological or personality defect or a personality disorder. In the fifth edition of the *Diagnostic and Statistical Manual of Mental Disorders* (DSM-5; American Psychiatric Association 2013), the condition was renamed and clarified. Gender dysphoria is a condition that arises from the incongruence between an individual's experienced gender and assigned gender, and symptoms of gender dysphoria improve when individuals are able to live in their experienced gender. In Western Europe and the United States, prevalence of gender dysphoria ranges between 0.001% and 0.002% (Judge et al. 2014; Landén et al. 1996; van Kesteren et al. 1996).

## GENDER AFFIRMATION TREATMENTS

Transgender individuals with gender dysphoria sometimes seek gender affirmation therapies to match their experienced (identified) gender with their biological (assigned) gender—although not everyone with gender dysphoria or a transgender identity will want these medical treatments. These therapies include hormone replacement therapy (HRT) (testosterone blockers, estrogen and progesterone, and testosterone) and gender-affirming procedures, which include reconstructive surgeries (vaginoplasty, phalloplasty, mastectomy, breast implants, facial reconstruction) and nonsurgical procedures (e.g., laser hair removal, voice training). The highly individualized process of gender affirmation therapies can be lengthy—in some cases, it can take up to several years. Therefore, transgender individuals with gender dysphoria present with unique challenges that require a multidisciplinary approach to treatment. World Professional Association for Transgender Health (WPATH) provides guidelines for assessment and treatment of gender dysphoria and guidelines to safely initiate gender affirmation therapies (World Professional Association for Transgender Health 2011).

HRT, which is a common first step in the gender affirmation process, is managed by clinicians (endocrinologists, primary care physicians, and psychiatrists) and is individualized depending on the individual's comfort level in gender expression and underlying health status. Current WPATH guidelines require individuals to have the capacity to give written informed consent and an absence of medical conditions that would prevent them from receiving hormonal treatments (World Professional Association for Transgender Health 2011). For surgical procedures, current WPATH guidelines require individuals to have been receiving HRT for at least 12 months and to provide two letters from two different mental health providers (World Professional Association for Transgender Health 2011), although these guidelines are becoming less restrictive over time. Requirements are also different depending on the specific surgical procedure. WPATH Standards of Care 8 will be published in 2020, and it has been proposed that gender affirmation surgery requirements be changed in these new guidelines.

## A NOTE ON DIAGNOSIS

Although *gender dysphoria* is used multiple times in this chapter, it should be noted that the diagnosis remains controversial. Just as homosexuality was removed from DSM in 1973, many proponents of transgender rights believe gender dysphoria does not belong in DSM as a mental disorder. It is believed that variants in gender identity, just like sexual orientation, are part of normal human expression. This diagnosis and history of treatment have caused tension between mental health care providers and transgender patients. Transgender individuals are often concerned with being pathologized for their gender identity and might avoid mental health treatment altogether out of fear a clinician might try to "cure" them of their gender diversity. Clinicians should keep this in mind when working with transgender individuals and be respectful of a person's individual beliefs about the subject.

# Questions Well-Meaning People Ask

### How do I find out if a patient is transgender?

There is no way of knowing if somebody is transgender without actually asking them about their gender identity. The best way to approach this is to develop a habit of beginning each new patient evaluation by going over some basic demographic information, including gender identity. Some electronic medical record systems now have a section that shows the patient's gender identity and preferred pronouns in addition to the assigned sex at birth; however, given the possibility of errors and misrepresentation, it is still a better practice to ask the patient directly.

### How do I know what pronouns to use? The patient's preferred name? Sexual orientation?

Similar to gender identity, there is no way of knowing someone's preferred gender pronouns. preferred name, or sexual orientation without actually asking openly. It is also important to remember that medical records can misrepresent any or all of this information, and these things can change over time. One common mistake many clinicians make is to look at the patient's gender identity and presentation and make an assumption as to what gender pronouns they might be using. The best approach is to ask the patient directly.

### Why is it important to know that someone is transgender?

Transgender people are present in everyday life, and not knowing a patient's gender identity can lead to some medical and ethical mistakes. For example, not counseling an FTM patient, who might still have female reproductive organs, about birth control might lead to issues that would not be present for a cisgender male, such as unaddressed pregnancy risks and/or potential medication side effects and risks. Moreover, not knowing a patient's gender identity prevents the clinician from understanding patients fully, including their psychosocial stressors, leading to poor patient care and doctor-patient relationship.

### Are there any biological underpinnings of transgender identity?

This is a very complex area, and the research in this area is quite limited; however, a few neuroimaging studies (Garcia-Falgueras and Swaab 2008; Kruijver et al. 2000; Zhou et al.

1995) have investigated the transgender brain from functional and anatomical standpoints and compared it with the cisgender brain. These studies show that there are functional and structural resemblances between the transgender brain and its identified gender, even prior to the initiation of HRT, suggesting that there might be some biological underpinnings of gender in the brain. However, it is important to note that many of these findings are inconsistent

## What is the most common reason for a transgender individual to see a psychiatrist?

The most common reasons why transgender people are seen in an outpatient psychiatric setting are gender dysphoria and mood and anxiety disorders, including generalized anxiety disorder, major depressive disorder (MDD), posttraumatic stress disorder, and suicidal ideation. Gender dysphoria has some overlapping symptoms with other psychiatric conditions, such as mood disorders (e.g., dysphoric mood), and, when not treated adequately, it can lead to depression, significant decrease in and disruption of overall functionality, and poor gender transition outcomes. Likewise, when comorbid psychiatric conditions are not treated adequately, they can have a negative effect on a transgender individual's overall quality of life and affect the overall flow of gender transition. Although gender dysphoric symptoms might be present in a transgender person's life, it is important for clinicians to be mindful not to miss major psychiatric symptoms that could be present in any patient—depression, anxiety, mania, or psychosis.

In addition to treating gender dysphoria, the role of a psychiatrist in transgender care can be divided into several different areas: 1) treatment of the mood component of gender dysphoria through counseling, psychotherapy, and/or medication management; 2) assessing the patient for readiness for gender affirmation treatments such as HRT and gender affirmation surgeries; 3) monitoring and treating emotional side effects of HRT; 4) providing patients with letters of support for HRT and gender affirmation surgeries; 5) providing patients with documentation needed to change their legal name, gender markers, and birth certificates; 6) referring patients to appropriate medical specialists (e.g., endocrinology, surgery); and 7) working with the nonphysician support team (nurses, social workers, psychologists, case managers, nurse practitioners, and physician assistants) to provide comprehensive care.

**What are some of the most common comorbidities in transgender mental health care?**

The most common psychiatric problems transgender people present with are mood disorders (MDD and anxiety disorders), followed by substance abuse. Etiology of mood disorders in the transgender population might be multifactorial: 1) untreated gender dysphoria; 2) poor socioeconomic status and discrimination, leading to less access to health care, which results in worsening in physical and mental health; 3) undiagnosed gender dysphoria misdiagnosed as MDD; and 4) some internal factors such as internalized transphobia. Bockting describes internalized transphobia as discomfort with one's identity stemming from societal gender expectations (Bockting 2015).

In addition, it is important to mention the concept of minority stress. Meyer's sexual minority stress model (Meyer 2003) describes external factors and internal factors (e.g., internalized transphobia, pessimism, nondisclosure of sexual orientation) related to an individual's minority status that have an impact on mental health status and resilience. This concept influenced researchers to develop a more gender-specific model, the gender minority stress model (Testa et al. 2015). Further research in this area (Testa et al. 2017) showed that victimization and discrimination leading to mental stress is strongly correlated with suicidality.

In the current literature, there are a number of studies showing the effects of external stressors on mood disorders in the transgender population, but research on internal factors leading to mood disorders and suicidality is scarce. Mood disorders and suicidality in the transgender population are more complicated than a linear correlation between gender-related external and internal stress leading to mood disorders and suicidality. To date, there are no published studies identifying clear predictors for suicide attempts in this population.

**Which specialties are involved in comprehensive transgender care?**

For most transgender people, primary care physicians, psychiatrists, or internal medicine doctors are responsible for transgender care and provide general medical care in addition to nonsurgical gender affirmation–specific care. In specialized academic institutions, these responsibilities are divided among specialists. In addition to a psychiatrist who provides mental health care and clearance for gender affirmation treatments, the team includes a primary care physician or an endocrinologist who can initiate and monitor HRT; surgeons (uro-gynecologist/ob-gyn, general surgeon, plastic surgeon) who can provide vaginoplasty, phalloplasty, hysterectomy, mastectomy, and facial feminization surgeries; a social worker who can help with coordination of care and access to clinical and social resources and legal help with changing legal name, gender markers, and birth certificates; a psychologist for counseling; and a transgender clinic team coordinator who makes sure that all of the visits happen in a timely and efficient manner.

**What is the right age to start HRT? What are some of the common practices for minors?**

Clinicians can provide cross-sex hormones for medical transition for people who are 18 years and older and have no contraindications (serious medical and psychiatric comorbidities). Per WPATH guidelines, patients do not need psychiatric clearance; however, they need to be made aware of the risks and benefits of starting HRT and sign a consent form. For people who are 18 years and older, parental consent is needed in order to start HRT. For gender-nonconforming prepubescent children, the general approach by experienced clinicians is to use puberty blockers (gonadotropin-releasing hormone analogues) to slow down and stop puberty and prevent secondary sexual characteristics from occurring until the gender identity matures and stabilizes and/or until the individual is older than 18 and can consent for the procedures. Some outpatient LGBT clinics in the United States start HRT with minors on a case-by-case basis, depending on the severity of gender dysphoria and the stability of the gender identity and the psychosocial stability of the individual.

**What are some of the effects and side effects of HRT?**

The main goal behind starting HRT is to achieve the secondary sex characteristics of the identified gender. For MTF individuals, female hormones (estrogen and progesterone) are usually not enough to achieve the desired feminizing effects. Therefore, HRT usually starts with testosterone blockade (spironolactone) followed by feminizing hormones (estrogens and/or progesterone). These hormones lead to softening of the skin, redistribution of body fat, lessening of body hair, breast growth, and shrinkage of male genitalia. For some MTF individuals with male-type baldness, finasteride, which acts on hair cells and blocks testosterone's hair-reducing effects, is also beneficial. Feminizing hormones increase coagulability, therefore increasing the risk of deep vein thrombosis. This risk is further increased in smokers.

For FTM individuals, testosterone monotherapy provides sufficient masculinization and leads to clitoral enlargement, body fat redistribution, increase in muscle mass, increase in body hair, male-type baldness, and deepening of the voice. Side effects include increased risk for osteopenia. Results of studies on whether or not testosterone can undo the protective effects of estrogens on cardiovascular health (e.g., Unger 2016) are not very clear.

**What are the contraindications for HRT?**

There are no absolute contraindications for HRT; however, clinicians have to be aware of certain medical conditions that might require extra attention, and prescribing sex hormones in those situations could result in complications. For example, for a patient with a history of breast cancer estrogen would be contraindicated. Another condition for which there is a relative contraindication for using estrogens is hypercoagulability. If the patient has an underlying medical condition that causes hypercoagulability, or if the patient develops deep vein thrombosis (DVT) while taking estrogen, the estrogen should be stopped, and the patient should receive treatment for the DVT. In some cases, restarting estrogens may be possible under the guidance of a hematologist. In addition, patients should be counseled about drug-drug interactions and other conditions (e.g., smoking) that could increase the risk for DVT risk. For testosterone replacement, clinicians need to screen patients for hyperlipidemia, polycythemia, and liver disease, although none of these conditions is an absolute contraindication.

In addition to medical side effects and/or contraindications, clinicians should also continue screening for mood and anxiety issues during the initiation and maintenance phases of HRT use. Although not all patients experience mood changes with HRT, some patients describe some mood instability, anxiety, and irritability while taking HRT, which is often referred to by patients as "going through a second puberty." Psychiatrists should be aware of these effects and screen for mood, anxiety, and irritability at every session. An example of a difficult clinical decision regarding starting or continuing HRT is severe gender dysphoria and severe comorbid MDD that may be affecting all areas of the patient's life that will not get better without help from HRT. In such a scenario, HRT could be started with close monitoring and plans to stop HRT if the underlying conditions (depression, impulsivity, anger outbursts) are worsened by the hormone treatment.

### Is certification needed and available for psychiatrists to treat TG people?

Currently, there are no mandatory requirements for psychiatrists prior to treating transgender people. However, WPATH offers training and certification for all providers throughout the year.

### What are some of the legal hurdles transgender individuals must go through?

There are several legal matters that transgender people might have to deal with, such as legal name change, changing gender markers on identification and/or driver's licenses, and changing birth certificates and identifiers in the medical records. The complexity of these procedures changes from state to state, and not all of these options are available in all states. For instance, some states allow name change and changing gender markers but do not allow any changes on the original birth certificate, which can cause discrepancies between the patient's documents. In addition, these changes can also lead to lapses in medical coverage.

### What can be expected after gender affirmation surgeries?

Some clinicians and patients see gender affirmation surgery as the ultimate solution to or cure for gender dysphoria or the ultimate final step of transition. Although this may be true for some patients, for others it is not. For some patients, after having spent years (and sometimes decades) with gender dysphoria and the psychosocial issues that stem from it, it might be very difficult to adjust to a new life. Sometimes, gender dysphoria persists even after transition goals have been achieved, and long-term therapy is required to address these issues. In addition, some gender affirmation surgeries have long and complicated recovery periods, with vaginoplasty and phalloplasty surgeries being the most complicated and most difficult. Vaginoplasty is followed by a 4- to 6-week recovery period, after which patients must start dilating the neovagina to avoid atresia of the new tissue. For phalloplasty, preparation and recovery take even longer. The patient must first undergo surgery to create a tissue flap (from the forearm or thigh area), which is used to build the neophallus. The patient then undergoes a series of operations to shape the neophallus, and, depending on the approach, to implant an erectile apparatus. Patients require significant psychiatric and emotional support during and after these procedures.

# Themes That May Emerge in Therapy

Each transgender patient is unique and presents with unique challenges and questions, however, certain themes emerge in transgender care. These themes are outlined in the following subsections.

## HEALTH DISPARITIES

The Institute of Medicine reports that LGBTQ+ people, especially transgender people, have less access to health care, which leads to poorer overall health, higher rates of substance abuse, mood disorders (depression and anxiety disorders), and suicide. Past surveys of medical professionals reveal that physicians do not feel comfortable or knowledgeable enough to treat LGBTQ+ patients, especially transgender people (AMA GLMA Physician Survey 2009; Eliason et al. 2011). In the 2011 National Transgender Discrimination Study, 19% of transgender people surveyed reported that they were refused medical care because of their transgender or gender-nonconforming status, and 50% reported having to teach their medical providers about transgender care (Grant et al. 2011). Many reported postponing medical care because of discrimination (28%) or inability to afford care (48%). These issues and their health outcomes are common themes that emerge in transgender care.

## AGING

Aging is a difficult and sometimes existential problem for many individuals regardless of their gender identity and sexual orientation, but it becomes an even bigger issue in the transgender population. With aging come medical problems, and for transgender individuals who have not gone through medical or surgical transition, these medical issues can present unique challenges, such as contraindications for HRT and/or gender affirmation surgeries. Most transgender people have a difficult time finding acceptance in their families and end up having to separate themselves from their biological families. For such patients, aging can be a difficult and isolating process, especially if they were not able to build their own families and/or friend circles—their families of choice.

## COMING OUT

Although not all transgender people come out, coming out is one of the most important topics in transgender mental health care and can be a recurrent topic of conversation in a psychiatric setting. In the transgender experience, coming out can be a longitudinal, multistep process rather than a one-time event. There are several reasons why the coming-out process can be complex.

1. When it comes to gender-nonconforming youth (<18 years), 80% of this population mature to have a cisgender identity with a homosexual or bisexual orientation. This statistic has recently been challenged, and long-term outcomes of gender atypical children are still being investigated.
2. Some transgender people experience confusion between sexual orientation and gender identity during the earlier phases of gender identity exploration. Especially in rural, less educated areas, where there is no exposure to sexual and gender minorities, it might be very difficult for a transgender individual to understand the internal processes leading to a mature gender identity and sexual orientation. In such cases, that individual may come out as gay, lesbian, or bisexual, but as the exploration continues, it becomes more apparent that the main source of the dysphoria is the mismatch between the body and the identified gender but not necessarily the person's sexual orientation (although transgender people can have heterosexual, homosexual, pansexual, or asexual orientation, regardless of their gender identity).
3. In some cases, sexual orientation matures before the gender identity does. In these cases, the individual comes out as gay, lesbian, or bisexual but discovers later on that they also have gender dysphoria, which leads to coming out as transgender later in life.

Coming out is an important part of the conversation in a psychiatric setting because it affects the person's quality of the life as well as their safety and sometimes readiness for gender affirmation treatments. For example, a transgender individual who is financially dependent on their family may have a very difficult time coming out to their family if there is a risk of abandonment and/or a threat to their safety. Inevitably, this affects or delays the individual's gender affirmation treatments and gender-congruent expression.

Coming out is not a one-dimensional process. Transgender people (LGBTQ+ people in general, for that matter) come out in more than one area in their lives in order to live more authentic lives: a transgender person may be fully out in their social circle and family but might be in the closet in their work environment because of various reasons such as job security. This process affects the overall quality of life and the course of the gender affirmation treatments, and the effects of coming out need to be assessed at each psychiatric visit to ensure patient safety and quality of life.

## COMMUNITY

Community is very important in transgender mental health care and could have a big impact on patients' lives. As mentioned in the subsection "Coming Out," the transgender experience can be an isolating and confusing experience, especially in rural parts of the world, and a transgender individual can have the perception that they are the only person having this experience. It is therefore of great importance for transgender individuals to be connected to their community for support. The community does not necessarily have to be an LGBTQ+ community, but it is often very important for the transgender individual to have friends who are LGBTQ+ or who are going through gender transition because the transition can be very challenging physically and emotionally, and having someone who has been through these phases and/or who can understand and give emotional support can improve the transition significantly.

## DATING

Although dating is not the main focus of the psychiatric interview, it is a common topic that comes up, and it can be very informative as to the patient's transition status, physical and emotional maturity, and sexual orientation. In addition, dating can be a window into the psychological and emotional development of the transgender individual.

1. In contrast with their cisgender and straight counterparts, transgender individuals may have a very difficult time dating before, during, and after transition; therefore, transgender individuals may have issues with stability in their dating lives longer than cisgender individuals do.
2. Considering gender identity and sexual orientation as fluctuating or evolving phenomena that mature over a long period, an individual's dating could be an indicator of their gender identity and orientation.
3. Dating can be a source of distress for some individuals because dating and sex often come with their own challenges when it comes to the transgender experience. For instance, a transgender female (MTF) individual who has not had vaginoplasty might find herself in the difficult position of not being able to experience penetrative vaginal sex, which could affect her relationship with her sexual partners as well her overall satisfaction.

## FAMILY

Similar to dating, family life can be an indicator of or window into the patient's readiness for gender transition and/or gender expression as well as coming out and therefore constitutes an important part of the psychiatric interview. Family is a very common theme that emerges in transgender care. Regardless of the patient's age, gender, and transition status, family is one of the most important areas in a transgender person's life. For transgender youth, family is vital. Not only is the family the main source of safety, shelter, and financial stability, but for minors family support is crucial and at times is a must, especially when it comes to gender transition procedures such as puberty blocking, cross-sex hormones, and gender affirmation surgeries. For young individuals older than 18 years, family may still be the main source of emotional and financial support.

For older transgender patients, family can be important for other reasons: older transgender individuals who have started a family of their own while still in the closet may have a very difficult time. The risk of losing family support and concerns about the spouse's reaction may prevent individuals from coming out and cause them to delay or cancel gender affirmation treatments. Severing family ties can result in significant financial and emotional burden and isolation. Starting a family during or after the transition can be challenging as well—from difficulties in finding a life partner to issues related to conception and emotional problems during transition.

In addition to biological/assigned family, chosen family (family of choice) is also very important in a transgender person's life. In many ways, chosen families can be a great source of support and stability in a transgender person's life, and given that chosen family may consist of individuals who identify as LGBTQ+, the connection and the level of understanding within a chosen family can be much deeper than within a biological family.

## FINANCES

Health disparities, discrimination, and lack of job security lead transgender individuals to have a low socioeconomic status. Financial instability can be stressful in and of itself, and not having a stable income, health insurance, or access to transgender-competent health care can also have some significant negative effects on transgender mental health: some gender affirmation treatments (e.g., laser hair removal, vaginoplasty) are not covered by insurance, and without health insurance, it may be impossible for transgender individuals to afford regular doctor visits, hormonal treatments, and surgical procedures. Transgender people thus may end up having to delay crucial treatments such as gender affirmation surgeries. Without gender affirmation treatments, gender dysphoria does not improve, and it will continue to affect transgender individuals' lives on a daily basis. Moreover, when not treated, gender dysphoria can lead to MDD, complicating the picture and having potentially fatal consequences, especially considering that transgender people are already at higher risk for mood disorders and suicide (à Campo et al. 2003; Dhejne et al. 2011; Hepp et al. 2005; Heylens et al. 2014). It is very important to note that when patients are not given access to treatments or when their health care needs are not met by health care professionals, they might seek these things elsewhere—such as ordering hormones off the Internet and sharing needles for hormone injections.

## HIV AND AIDS

Closely related to health disparities and socioeconomic status, transgender people have been shown to have poorer overall health and higher rates of sexually transmitted diseases, including HIV (Gay and Lesbian Medical Association 2001; Ward et al. 2014). It is therefore crucial for clinicians to discuss these issues. Moreover, given the complexity and variety of sexual practices and anatomies when it comes to transgender people, it is very important to make sexual history part of the general psychiatric assessment.

## LEGAL ISSUES

The most common legal issues that come up in transgender care are issues related to legal name changes, changing gender markers on driver's licenses, and changing birth certificates. In most states, changing the legal name and gender markers are relatively easier procedures, although given that both procedures require application and/or processing fees, they may be difficult for some transgender individuals who are too young and/or who do not have the financial means to take care of these procedures. Changing the birth certificate might be a bigger issue, depending on the state. Some states do not allow birth certificates to be altered, which creates discrepancies in individuals' records. Another layer of complexity around this issue involves medical records and health insurance. In states where patients are not allowed to change their birth certificates, it might also be difficult to change the gender markers in their medical records and/or insurance information, which can lead to problems in the patients' health care.

## MENTAL HEALTH AND ILLNESS

Mental health and illness are essential topics in transgender mental health. Most transgender people struggle with gender dysphoria, often for years, before seeing a mental health provider. For individuals in bigger cities with more resources and better access to mental health care, outreach programs, and a well-rooted LGBTQ+ community, issues such as gender dysphoria can be addressed sooner, and transgender individuals can get the help they need and get connected with resources. In more rural areas, however, it might be very difficult for transgender people to find health care providers who understand the root of the problem and to get much-needed help. Untrained clinicians often confuse gender dysphoria with mood disorders such as depression and anxiety disorders.

Moreover, there might be an assumption among the general public and untrained clinicians that being transgender and/or having gender dysphoria unequivocally means an individual also has depression. However, research shows that when transgender people with gender dysphoria get the gender affirmation treatments they need, gender dysphoria improves, and retrospective analysis of these individuals shows that gender dysphoria was not associated with other comorbid psychiatric diagnoses, suggesting that only a subset of transgender people diagnosed with mood disorders in the earlier, pre-HRT phase of their transition actually had gender dysphoria (Heylens et al. 2014). That said, LGBTQ+ people and transgender people in particular are still considered to be at high risk for mood disorders and suicide, which makes it an imperative to talk about mental health during each outpatient visit.

## INTERSECTIONALITY

The term *intersectionality* refers to the idea that all human beings have multiple layers of complex identities (sex, gender, race, health status, socioeconomic status, nationality, and many others) and that these identities all interact with each other, contributing to and creating an individual's unique presentation in the world. Thinking of and seeing transgender individuals this way not only enriches the doctor-patient relationship but also prevents generalizations and/or assumptions from happening.

## SEX

Sex is an important topic in a psychiatric interview with a transgender patient. Taking a sexual history at every visit (or at least doing so periodically) provides invaluable information and insight into the patient's sexual orientation, coming out status, and readiness for transition. In addition, reviewing a patient's sexual history is a safety measure, providing a means for understanding and preventing certain health risks such as unwanted pregnancy and sexually transmitted diseases (STDs). Assumptions about sexual orientation and sexual practices can lead to mistakes. For example, a masculine-presenting patient who enjoys penetrative vaginal sex could be at risk for pregnancy, and a female-presenting patient engaged in penile-anal sex should be screened for STDs by obtaining samples from all of the body surfaces involved in sex, including the penile mucosa.

## RELIGION AND SPIRITUALITY

Spirituality and religion are common themes that come up in transgender care. These concepts enter one's life very early and from a young age affect an individual's family culture, overall development, and view of the world. Considering that most transgender people spend their early formative years in the closet or trying to figure out their gender identity and/or sexual orientation, spirituality and religion also significantly affect their process of coming out or understanding their own identity. In families where there is a strict religious culture and a conservative narrative in which being transgender is considered a "sin," gender-nonconforming kids grow up with the perception that their feelings are sinful and their identity is unacceptable. Growing up in such an environment can lead to a major disconnect within the individual, leading to self-hatred and depression. On the other hand, if spirituality brings acceptance and openness, it can lead to self-discovery, a much smoother transition, and acceptance. Transgender people with strong religious beliefs and upbringing usually struggle between accepting their own identity and accepting the religious doctrine in which they believe.

## TRANSFERENCE AND COUNTERTRANSFERENCE

Transference and countertransference are important phenomena in any psychiatric interview, but they become even more important when it comes to transgender care because of the unique role a psychiatrist plays. Because one of the responsibilities of the psychiatrist is to assess for readiness for gender affirmation treatments and to provide patients with letters of recommendation when they are deemed ready, psychiatrists can often be seen as "gatekeepers" or "roadblocks," which could affect the doctor-patient relationship in a negative way, preventing transgender people from being completely open with their psychiatrist and potentially leading to poor treatment outcomes and high dropout rates. Explaining the role of the psychiatrist and clarifying the steps that lead to gender affirmation treatments, including side effects and adverse events associated with these treatments (which could prolong or interrupt the transition period), could potentially prevent these negative outcomes. Moreover, there is also a history in medicine of seeing gender dysphoria as a pathology, and attempts have been made at conversion therapy. As a result, patients might be afraid a psychiatrist will attempt to change their identity. Understanding these fears and starting the doctor-patient relationship with openness and by setting up clear expectations are crucial in transgender care.

## Conclusion

Approaching transgender patients in a nonassuming, non-judgmental way and starting with open-ended questions is the key to building relationships. The initial evaluation of a transgender person includes a full gender development evaluation, a full psychiatric evaluation with screening for gender dysphoria, and, if needed, an assessment of readiness for certain gender affirmation treatments (e.g., hormone replacement therapies, gender affirmation surgeries).

In order to fully evaluate for readiness, psychosocial determinants, coming out status, and the patient's support system need to be assessed at every visit to prevent future mistakes or rushed decisions. The patient's multilayered identity (also known as intersectionality), which includes all areas in a person's life (nationality, socioeconomic status, health status, race, dating status, and many others) should be taken into consideration. The patient should be viewed as a whole rather than a single layer of identity such as their transgender identity.

Clinically, LGBTQ+ people, especially transgender people, are at high risk for mood and anxiety disorders. At the same time, symptoms of gender dysphoria may be confused with symptoms of major depressive disorder; therefore, being always alert about the possibility of gender dysphoria can prevent mistakes.

# FIVE TAKE-HOME POINTS

- Starting the psychiatric interview with open-ended questions and going over gender identity, sexual orientation, and preferred name and pronouns can prevent mistakes and assumptions and help start a good foundation in transgender care.

- Patients come to psychiatric appointments with fear of judgment and criticism. Laying out the purpose of the visit and being open and honest can help ease the tension and fear that patients may be experiencing and is a good first step in building relationships.

- In addition to a detailed history of current and past psychiatric comorbidities, assessing psychosocial stressors, sexual history, coming out status, and occupational history can provide invaluable information regarding the patient's readiness for gender affirmation treatments.

- Gender dysphoria is a condition stemming from a mismatch between assigned and identified gender. Because its overlapping symptoms with mood disorders (depression and anxiety) can be confusing to untrained clinicians, it is important to separate the two in order to provide the best treatment and guidance for patients.

- Screening patients for HRT side effects and comorbid psychiatric issues that are common in the transgender community (mood and anxiety disorders, suicidality, substance abuse) can lead to early capture of some of these issues and prevention of complications.

## Resources

American Academy of Family Physicians: Recommended Curriculum Guidelines for Family Medicine Residents: Lesbian, Gay, Bisexual, Transgender Health (1AAFP Reprint No 289D), August 2016. www.aafp.org/dam/AAFP/documents/medical_education_residency/program_directors/Reprint289D_LGBT.pdf

Association of American Medical Colleges: AAMC Videos and Resources about LGBT Health and Health Care, avaialble at www.aamc.org/what-we-do/mission-areas/diversity-inclusion/lgbt-health-resources/videos

World Professional Association for Transgender Health (WPATH), www.wpath.org

## References

à Campo J, Nijman H, Merckelbach H, Evers C: Psychiatric comorbidity of gender identity disorders: a survey among Dutch psychiatrists. Am J Psychiatry 160(7):1332–1336, 2003 12832250

American Psychiatric Association: Diagnostic and Statistical Manual of Mental Disorders, 5th Edition. Arlington, VA, American Psychiatric Association, 2013

Bockting W: Internalized transphobia, in The International Encyclopedia of Human Sexuality. Edited by Whelehan P, Bolin A. Hoboken, NJ, Wiley-Blackwell, 2015, pp 583–625

Dhejne C, Lichtenstein P, Boman M, et al: Long-term follow-up of transsexual persons undergoing sex reassignment surgery: cohort study in Sweden. PLoS One 6(2):e16885, 2011 21364939

Eliason MJ, Dibble SL, Robertson PA: Lesbian, gay, bisexual, and transgender (LGBT) physicians' experiences in the workplace. J Homosex 58:(10)1355–1371, 2011 22029561

Garcia-Falgueras A, Swaab DF: A sex difference in the hypothalamic uncinate nucleus: relationship to gender identity. Brain 131(pt 12):3132–3146, 2008 18980961

Gay and Lesbian Medical Association: Healthy People 2010: a companion document for lesbian, gay, bisexual, and transgender (LGBT) health. San Francisco, CA, Gay and Lesbian Medical Association, 2001

Grant JM, Mottet LA, Tanis J, et al: Injustice at every turn: A report of the National Transgender Discrimination Survey. Washington, DC, National Center for Transgender Equality and the National Gay and Lesbian Task Force, 2011

Hepp U, Kraemer B, Schnyder U: Psychiatric comorbidity in gender identity disorder. J Psychosom Res 58(3):259–261, 2005 15865950

Heylens G, Elaut E, Kreukels BP, et al: Psychiatric characteristics in transsexual individuals: multicentre study in four European countries. Br J Psychiatry 204(2):151–156, 2014 23869030

Judge C, O'Donovan C, Callaghan G, et al: Gender dysphoria: prevalence and co-morbidities in an Irish adult population. Front Endocrinol (Lausanne) 5:87, 2014 24982651

Kinsey AC, Pomeroy WR, Martin CE: Sexual behavior in the human male. Am J Public Health 93(6):894–898, 2003

Klein F, Sepekoff B, Wolf TJ: Sexual orientation: a multi-variable dynamic process. J Homosex 11(1–2):35–49, 1985 4056393

Kruijver FP, Zhou JN, Pool CW, et al: Male-to-female transsexuals have female neuron numbers in a limbic nucleus. J Clin Endocrinol Metab 85(5):2034–2041, 2000 10843193

Landén M, Wålinder J, Lundström B: Prevalence, incidence and sex ratio of transsexualism. Acta Psychiatr Scand 93(4):221–223, 1996 8712018

Meyer IH: Prejudice, social stress, and mental health in lesbian, gay, and bisexual populations: conceptual issues and research evidence. Psychol Bull 129(5):674–697, 2003 12956539

Meyer-Bahlburg HFL: From mental disorder to iatrogenic hypogonadism: dilemmas in conceptualizing gender identity variants as psychiatric conditions. Arch Sex Behav 39(2):461–476, 2010 19851856

Testa RJ, Habarth J, Peta J: Development of the gender minority stress and resilience measure. Psychol Sex Orientat Gend Divers 2(1):65–77, 2015

Testa RJ, Michaels MS, Bliss W, et al: Suicidal ideation in transgender people: gender minority stress and interpersonal theory factors. J Abnorm Psychol 126(1):125–136, 2017 27831708

Unger CA: Hormone therapy for transgender patients. Transl Androl Urol 5(6):877–884, 2016 28078219

van Kesteren PJ, Gooren LJ, Megens JA: An epidemiological and demographic study of transsexuals in The Netherlands. Arch Sex Behav 25(6):589–600, 1996 8931882

Ward BW, Dahlhamer JM, Galinsky AM, Joesti SS: Sexual orientation and health among U.S. adults: National Health Interview Survey, Natl Health Stat Report 15(77):1–10, 2014 25025690

World Professional Association for Transgender Health: Standards of Care for the Health of Transsexual, Transgender, and Gender Nonconforming People, 7th version. East Dundee, Illinois, World Professional Association for Transgender Health, 2011

Zhou JN, Hofman MA, Gooren LJ, Swaab DF: A sex difference in the human brain and its relation to transsexuality. Nature 378(6552):68–70, 1995 7477289

# Chapter 5

# Queer

## The First Q in LGBTQ²IAPA

SAM MARCUS, M.A.
E.K. BREITKOPF, M.A.

…[Q]ueers have always lived in the realm of the impossible.

*Alok Vaid-Menon (2018; they/them/their)*

## Psychological and Cultural Context

Queer is about more than sexual orientation; for many people, it is a politically charged identity that signals their resistance to heteronormativity. Historically, the term *queer* was used as a homophobic slur that contributed to violence against nonheterosexual people. Its reappropriation from a derogatory term to an empowering one began during the AIDS crisis in the late 1980s, when nonheterosexual activists stood in social and political opposition to heterosexist culture (Stryker 2017). At the time, President Reagan's administration was tragically slow in providing resources to fight the dramatically increasing number of people dying from HIV/AIDS-related illnesses (Shilts 1987/2011). By reclaiming the word queer, activists harnessed the shock value of the word's derogatory history and transformed it into a symbol of power and political resistance. Queer Nation, an antiviolence organization founded in 1990 by HIV/AIDS activists from ACT UP, proudly reclaimed *queer* as they chanted, "We're here! We're queer! Get used to it!" (Cava 2014). Today, queer is often used as an umbrella term to refer to the entire LGBTQ+ community in addition to being an individual identity. In this chapter, we focus on the latter, providing an introduction to what it means to identify as queer.

The term queer, as many folks use it today, was born out of resistance against homophobia and heteronormative oppression. Heteronormativity is a system of thought that perpetuates the belief that heterosexuality is normal and queerness is pathological (Kelly 2014). It manifests interpersonally, institutionally, socially, and politically after being socialized into our cultural frameworks from a very young age, promoting homophobia and reinforcing systematic and interpersonal oppression of queer people (for example, there is no need for a *Pocket Guide to Heterosexual Mental Health* because heterosexuality has never been treated as being sinful, perverse, or a mental illness). Additionally, racism, classism, sexism, cisgenderism, ableism, colorism, ageism, and other systems of oppression disenfranchise some LGBTQ+ voices more than others, especially those who occupy intersecting disempowered social positions (Combahee River Collective 1977/2000; Crenshaw 1989; Moradi 2017).

There is no one way of being queer. In fact, this is an important underpinning of the concept of queerness today. For many people, it is a constant state of becoming that resists linear, categorized, and static conceptualizations of life and of desire. The term works to disrupt the notion that human sexuality can be easily categorized (Butler 2004b) and that an individual's sexual identity is static and unchanging over the course of their life.

*Queer* also signals that gender is not a fundamental aspect of desire. Whereas *gay* and *lesbian* denote the gender identity of both the subject and the object of attraction (i.e., lesbian is understood to refer to a person who identifies as a woman who is attracted to other people who identify as women), queer sexuality does not require gender to be a major factor in the experience of attraction. This is similar to the term pansexual, which is often used by individuals who do not "see gender" in those they love and desire. *Pansexual* and *omnisexual* are both used by individuals who are attracted to all genders. The important difference lies in the attention paid to gender: many omnisexual people *do* see gender, whereas pansexual individuals do not. In this sense, a queer identity communicates that someone does not identify as heterosexual without identifying their gender or the genders of the people they desire. (Note that the term *heterosexual* is preferable to *straight* because of straight's implication that hetero-sexuality is normal and other sexualities are abnormal or crooked.)

The gender neutrality of queer makes it especially mean-ingful for trans and nonbinary people because it can be used to resist the *cisnormativity* (the assumption that all people are cisgender) common in LGB identity terms. As cultural dis-courses of gender continue to shift, the term *bisexual* has be-come more complicated for some people because of increasing social awareness of more than two genders and a growing re-sistance to cisnormativity. Thus, terms such as omnisexual and queer have become helpful alternatives for individuals who experience attractions to multiple genders. Many people also use the term queer to mark their distance from *homonor-mativity*, the pressure to look or act in certain ways in order to be seen as "really" lesbian or "really" gay, which is common in mainstream gay and lesbian communities. Historically, individ-uals in these homonormative communities have prioritized as-similation into white cisheteronormative society (e.g., by getting married, having a family) over destabilizing the white cishetero-sexism that maintains inequity in its social systems and institu-tions (Duggan 2003).

Nonheterosexual people of color have historically been marginalized by dominant white gay and lesbian communi-ties in the United States. Many of the chapter headings in this book, including queer, are widely used terms popularized and legitimized by the most powerful LGBTQ+ community members—white, formally educated activists. Although many people of color do identify with the word queer, others are uncomfortable with it. Thus, communities of color have long developed terminologies to describe their identities and experiences that are not used by white people. For example, *Ag* or *aggressive* and *stud*, which are similar to *butch* (more common in white communities), are used primarily by black and Latinx (a gender-neutral alternative to Latina or Latino) people to describe someone assigned female at birth, usually lesbian-identified, with a masculine gender presentation who may be read as male. Some black people identify as *same gender loving*—rather than queer, lesbian, or gay—a term that originated in the black community in the 1990s and does not contain the whiteness embedded in other terms.

The term homosexuality is considered offensive by many people in the LGBTQ+ community because of its diagnostic history. Unfortunately, mental health practitioners have historically legitimized white heteronormative and heterosexist (as well as cisnormative and cissexist) systems of oppression through the *Diagnostic and Statistical Manual of Mental Disorders* (DSM). The first three editions of DSM (American Psychiatric Association 1952, 1968, 1980) all pathologized homosexuality in different ways, although the degree of pathologization decreased over time as people within and outside the field of psychiatry pushed back against these practices. This history contributes to social stigma that queer people still experience in daily life, to the overdiagnosis of LGBTQ+ individuals in mental health care, and to the prevalence of clinicians lacking LGBTQ+ cultural competence—all of which can make some queer people feel hesitant to seek mental health care (Platt et al. 2018). These barriers to health care are especially common in the trans community, an estimated 21% of whom identify as queer—queer was the most common sexual orientation listed by the 27,715 trans respondents in the 2015 U.S. Transgender Survey, followed by pansexual (18%); gay, lesbian, or same gender loving (16%); heterosexual (15%); bisexual (14%); and asexual (10%) (James et al. 2016, p. 59).

One form of resistance against these oppressive histories are efforts to *queer* clinical practice through education, discussion, and institutional restructuring. The act of queering challenges normative binary ways of thinking about the self and others, not only in relation to sexuality but also to other intersecting issues such as disability, race, and gender (Burnes and Stanley 2017). This could include using demographic forms that ask patients to describe their various identities in their own words (rather than checking a box), providing clearly marked gender-neutral restrooms, or attending workshops on queer identities that expand your understanding and awareness of human sexuality and social structures.

In the past few decades, the visibility of queer people has been growing in U.S. media. Queer public figures such as musician Janelle Monáe, actors Rowan Blanchard and Natalie Morales, writer Jacob Tobia, and artist Alok Vaid-Menon (quoted at the beginning of the chapter) have significant followings on social media and represent a diverse cross-section of queer voices influencing public discourse. As representations of queer solidarity and activism have become more accessible through the rise of social media, so have information and resources for queer youth and adults in need of support and community. Queer clinicians have long taken on the work of resisting harmful heteronormative practices in clinical spaces, whether through scholarship, by creating queer-centered spaces for patients, or by working to educate nonqueer colleagues about queer cultural competence. In this spirit, in the remainder of this chapter, we offer some resources for how you might begin to think of what you can do to better serve your queer patients. We will address common questions about queer people as well as themes that may come up in therapy with a queer person.

# Questions Well-Meaning People Ask

Below are examples of questions nonqueer people ask about queer people. These might be questions you have yourself, questions your colleagues have asked, or questions your patients might ask you as an expert on identity and human behavior.

## IDENTITY

### How should I use the word queer so that it's not derogatory?

*Queer* is an identity and should be used only in reference to people who identify as such. Using person-first language is respectful, as is using *queer* as an adjective rather than as a noun (e.g., it is appropriate to say, "I was speaking with a person who identifies as queer the other day" but not appropriate to say, "I was speaking with a queer the other day," the latter of which is dehumanizing).

### What is the difference between queer and gay, lesbian, or bisexual?

As was discussed in the section "Psychological and Cultural Context" earlier in this chapter, *queer* is more than a sexual orientation. For many people, an important aspect of queer identity is resisting different normative ways of being, including heteronormativity and homonormativity. Depending on the person, this might mean challenging dominant notions of relationships (e.g., marriage, monogamy), intimacy (e.g., via such practices as kink and BDSM; see subsection "Sexuality and Intimacy"), and/or kinship (e.g., by reconceptualizing familial structures). Although people who identify as gay, lesbian, or bisexual may also challenge these ideas, this is a fundamental aspect of queer identity for many people.

**Do queer people also identify as LGB?**

Queer people may or may not also identify as gay, lesbian, or bisexual. The only way to know how a person identifies is to ask them directly, "How do you identify in terms of your sexual orientation?"

## What is the difference between queer and transgender?

Generally speaking, the terms queer and transgender address two different facets of a person's identity: queer refers to a person's sexual orientation, whereas transgender refers to a person's gender identity. Sexual orientation describes who a person is or is not attracted to. Gender identity describes a person's subjective sense of belonging to a gender category (Stryker 2017). Queer people may identify as any gender.

However, life outside of the gender and gay/hetero binaries has always been an important part of queer identities. Queerness does not assume that a person's sexual orientation is necessarily tied to the relationship between their gender identity and the gender identity of the people to whom they are attracted. Many people who identify as queer are attracted to people of an array of different genders. Additionally, people of many different genders may identify as queer.

**Do queer people use different pronouns?**

They might. The only way to find out is to ask.

Just as heteronormativity is the conscious or unconscious belief that heterosexuality is the normal or default sexual orientation, cisnormativity is the conscious or unconscious belief that cisgender identities are the normal or default gender identities. An anti-cisnormative approach is to always introduce yourself with your name and pronouns and to ask the name and pronouns of everyone you meet (e.g., "Hello, Sally. My name is Dr. X, and my pronouns are they/them/their. What are your pronouns?"). Even if you think it is obvious what pronouns an individual uses, these assumptions are not always correct. Cisgender people can normalize the practice of asking for pronouns by offering their own first. This also prevents trans people from being othered and dehumanized as someone whose pronouns and genders are unintelligible (Butler 2004a).

**What if someone says they are queer but I am not convinced that they are?**

It is the mental health provider's responsibility to respect the language patients use to identify themselves. This is especially important because of the long history of mental health providers undermining LGBTQ+ individuals' self-determination by pathologizing their identities as mental illnesses. There are, of course, situations in which individuals' identities are unstable, but it is critical to not assume that all people who are questioning their sexual or gender identity are experiencing clinical identity disturbance. It is also important to remember that a patient experiencing clinical identity disturbance may *also* be LGBTQ+.

**How should I ask a queer person about their identity?**

Asking a simple, open-ended question, such as "How do you identify?" may be the best place to start. You can be more specific by asking "How do you identify your sexual orientation?" or "How do you identify your gender?" Closed-ended questions or statements that contain assumptions (e.g., "Are you gay?") can sometimes leave people feeling unseen or even judged.

## RELATIONSHIPS

**Who is the man/woman in a queer relationship?**

This question that may come to mind for some heterosexual people. Because heterosexual relationships have long been the organizing template for understanding how partners relate to one another, people often feel compelled to try to fit queer relationships into this framework. This is a form of heterosexism. If this question does come to mind with a queer patient, it is best to take a moment and reflect on what is behind it. There are a number of reasons one might feel compelled to ask this question. For instance, it might be coming from your own anxieties about not knowing how queer partners relate to one another, either sexually or more generally in a relationship. Queer resources such as this book can help with that. However, if you are interested in the general dynamics in the patient's relationship, it is better to ask that question directly (e.g., "Tell me about the dynamics of your relationship") instead of assuming a heteronormative lens.

## My patient is nonbinary and describes themself as femme. What does that mean?

Femme and masc are two queer identities that some people use to describe their gender presentation or experience of gender distinct from their gender identity. A person who identifies as masc is conveying that they express and/or experience their gender in a masculine way, and, similarly, a femme expresses their gender in a feminine way. A femme or masc identity is not tied to a person's gender identity, to traditional gender roles of masculinity and femininity, or to heteronormative relationship dynamics, which suggest that women should be feminine and men should be masculine in order to be attractive to one another. Instead, femme and masc are queer identities that subvert these cisheteronormative assumptions; femininity and masculinity are experienced as part of one's queerness.

## Should I ask a queer person who they're attracted to?

An important backdrop here is that there has been a long history of heterosexual people feeling anxious in the company of queer people because their sexuality seems "unclear." As with any question about a queer person's intimate life, it is important to give yourself a moment to reflect on its clinical relevance. Are you asking this question because it is important for the person's care or because you may feel uncomfortable not knowing the gender of the people they tend to be attracted to?

## How might queer families differ from heteronormative families?

The normative heterosexual family in the United States (the heteronormative family) consists of a cisgender male father who is married to a cisgender female mother; together they have cisgender heterosexual children. A queer family might mirror the heteronormative family except for the sexual orientations and gender identities of the parents, but it could also differ in a variety of other ways. The parents' relationship could be non-monogamous (see next question), there might be more than two parents, family members may not be biologically related, the parents might not assume that their children are heterosexual, and/or the children might feel more empowered and free to explore their gender and sexual identities. The parents may not have come out until later in life and may have been in heterosexual relationships prior to their queer one. In terms of the family's position in the social world, they might face discrimination in various environments, and queer parents might worry about their children being treated differently because of their family's queerness. One person recently told me they were non-monogamous.

**What does that mean?**

Dominant narratives in the United States assume that adults in "healthy" relationships are monogamous and are oriented on a linear path toward cohabitation and marriage, with a prohibition against having sexual or intimate experiences with anyone outside of the two-person relationship. Although some queer people certainly identify with this trajectory, other queer people have relationships in which they engage sexually and/or intimately with individuals outside of the relationship with consent from their partner or even have multiple partnerships. *Consensual non-monogamies* is an umbrella term that encompasses a variety of relationship structures and orientations for people who do not seek monogamous relationships (Hardy and Easton 2017; Taormino 2008). These individuals may identify as being in an open relationship or as being responsibly or ethically non-monogamous, polyamorous, poly partnered, monogamish, or simply non-monogamous (see the following two examples). Although some heterosexual people may be non-monogamous, this does not mean they identify as queer. Additionally, not all queer people identify as non-monogamous.

CASE EXAMPLE 1: AN OPEN RELATIONSHIP

Jay is a 30-year-old queer, nonbinary person (pronouns: they/them/their). They are in an open, non-monogamous relationship with their partner, Sandra, a 29-year-old queer, femme, cisgender woman (pronouns: she/her/her). Jay often struggles with being perceived as a cishet (cisgender heterosexual) man because of how people perceive them individually and how people perceive their relationship with Sandra. Jay and Sandra have cohabitated since graduating college. Together, they have discussed the boundaries of their relationship, and once a week they each go on a date with another person and, if they would like to, may hook up with them. On occasion, they also invite a third person to hook up with them together as a couple.

CASE EXAMPLE 2: A POLYAMOROUS RELATIONSHIP

Zara is a 35-year-old queer, polyamorous, trans woman (pronouns: she/her/her) who lives with her primary partner,

Kris, a cis woman, with whom she is raising a child. She also has two other femme partners and spends time with each of them weekly. Both of them are friends with Kris and are like family to her child. Zara works at a company that describes itself as "queer and trans inclusive," but she does not feel she can be open about her poly identity and her family structure and often worries about being outed to her coworkers.

## SEXUALITY AND INTIMACY

### How do queer people have sex?

First, there are as many ways to have queer sex as there are queer people in the world. Second, it is often inappropriate to ask queer people how they have sex. If the motivation for your question is to satisfy your own curiosity, it is probably not an appropriate question. Clinically speaking, it is only appropriate to ask a queer person about their sexual habits if you would do the same with a heterosexual patient in a similar clinical situation. The answer must be important and relevant to the treatment in order for the question to be appropriate. Otherwise, sexual practices should be brought up only by the patient. Although it might not be relevant to ask a patient directly about their sexual practices, it is helpful to be aware of what types of sexual and intimate experiences may come up in a clinical context (see case examples) so as to avoid pathologizing these experiences.

### My patient told me they're in the queer kink community. What does that mean?

For some queer people, the term queer encompasses BDSM and kink identities (Sprott and Benoit Hadcock 2018), including bondage (B), dominance and submission (D/s), sadomasochism (SM), fantasy, role-playing, fetish, and a number of other consensual intimate or sexual experiences in which there is an exchange of pain and/or power (Taormino 2012).

It can feel highly vulnerable for a patient to share their kink and BDSM identities with their psychiatrist, particularly because psychiatry and psychology have a long history of pathologizing these alternative sexual practices that still persists. Psychiatry's view of sexual sadism, for example, is primarily informed by data collected from individuals in forensic settings whose sadism coincides with nonconsensual sex or other crimes (Burnes et al. 2017). Unfortunately, current diagnostic categories under paraphilic disorders also include people who enjoy *consensual* practices of sadism or masochism, get turned on while role-playing as or dressing in clothing that is socially designated for a different gender, or who prefer to have sex while smoking a cigarette. If they feel psychological distress because they are not socially accepted for these practices because of kinkphobia in society, they would technically meet criteria for DSM-5 diagnosis of a paraphilic disorder. There is a growing body of literature on kink to help challenge common misconceptions that pathologize BDSM practitioners and practices (Burnes et al. 2017; Ortmann and Sprott 2013; Taormino 2012).

**My patient sometimes has bruises or cuts on their arm and recently disclosed to me that they're a "sub." What does that mean? Should I be concerned about abuse?**

When someone describes themself with a kink or BDSM term such as *sub*, it is important to not assume that this is abuse. Although abuse does happen within the kink community, bruises and other bodily marks are a common part of a sub-identified person's enjoyment, and it can be hurtful and shaming to assume that this is abuse. Many people who identify as subs or switches (meaning they switch roles between dominant and submissive) consent to receiving bruises on their body from their partner. As with any kink practice, a healthy D/s relationship requires a significant level of communication between partners in which they discuss consent and boundaries, use safe words with one another, and openly share their desires for what they want to happen between them during play. *Play* is a word used by many people in the kink and BDSM community to describe interactions between individuals that are openly discussed, planned, and carried out with mutual consent. People often plan "scenes" in which, for example, a submissive partner shares a desire for the dominant partner to engage in a certain act with them (which, as with this patient, may lead to marks on the body). Together, they might discuss what feels right for each play partner, plan a scene, and then carry it out. Signs of abuse in D/s relationships mirror signs of abuse in non-D/s relationships. If your patient shares that they did not consent or want to engage in the acts that caused their bruises, then you should assess for abuse.

### Do all queer people engage in kink or BDSM?

No. However, it is a common practice for queer people. It is not always experienced as a sexual practice and can offer a space for enjoyment, healing, and agency. Many queer and non-queer people alike experience consensual pain and/or domination as a form of pleasure and thus seek out partners and relationships that allow them to safely and consensually explore these aspects of pleasure.

If you do encounter a patient who is talking about their kink and BDSM identities, it is important to be supportive of the risk the patient is taking to share their experience with you and to normalize and honor people's consensual acts with their partners, even if they might feel out of the ordinary to the practitioner. Research suggests that BDSM-identified individuals feel more supported when practitioners are open to learning and reading more about BDSM, are open to talking about BDSM issues, and promote and understand safe consensual practices (Kolmes et al. 2006).

## Themes that May Emerge in Therapy

A number of themes may come up in therapy with a queer patient. These themes can also be complicated by the patient's other social identities and the social identities they might read from the therapist, which become part of the treatment.

### "IS MY THERAPIST QUEER?"

The question of self-disclosure with patients is always a complicated one but can be more complicated when working with historically marginalized groups (Levounis and Anson 2012). Queer people may wonder if a therapist is queer and may struggle with questions of whether the therapist is heterosexual, gay, lesbian, or bisexual. All of these identity categories carry meanings for the treatment that can, at times, make it difficult for a patient to open up and, at other times, make it easier to trust the therapist. If a patient begins to voice curiosity about these questions, it can be helpful to explore with a queer patient what it would mean for them to know or not know the therapist's sexual identity; make space for any thoughts and feelings that may come up in relation to the question; and think through, with the patient, how knowing may help or hinder their work together. Some people advocate for queer therapists working with queer patients to self-disclose so as to create a potentially more trusting context for their work; it is not necessary for a heterosexual therapist to disclose their heterosexuality because it is typically presumed. Disclosing heterosexuality to a queer patient who has not asked for the therapist's sexual orientation may feel offensive to the patient, as if the therapist is trying to distance themself from queerness.

## BEING "QUEER ENOUGH"

As with many marginalized people, queer people often struggle with their visibility as queer, feeling either "too much" or "not enough," which can cause feelings of loneliness, alienation, and anxiety. For instance, patients may share that they are struggling to become more visibly queer in some contexts while, at the same time, worrying that they will come off as "excessive" or may feel "exposed" in other contexts. This can be particularly true for people who are just beginning to identify themselves as queer and may not yet have queer friends or connections to the queer community.

A person who adheres to binary norms of gender, whether trans or cis, may struggle with feelings of insecurity about their queerness and feel a pull to identify exclusively with more binary terms such as lesbian, bisexual, gay, or heterosexual. Some struggle with wanting to be read as queer while in a relationship that may be read as heterosexual, such as a queer cis woman dating a cis man or a queer trans man dating a cis woman. This can be especially complicated as people navigate shifts in their gender identifications and expressions that impact their visibility as a queer person. For example, a trans/nonbinary person who decides to take testosterone may be uncomfortable when people begin to read them as cishet male; this person might experience anxiety about feeling as if they have to choose between being comfortable in their body and being visibly queer.

At the same time, many people may experience others reacting negatively to the potential unintelligibility that comes with being queer in non-queer spaces. This can significantly exacerbate anxieties about being excessive and/or seen and can intensify internalized queerphobia, or feelings of self-hatred rooted in discriminatory narratives about queer people.

## FEELING ALIENATED

The experience of alienation, or feeling different from others, is an important part of queer identity for many people and often shapes the childhoods of queer people. It can be a positive aspect of being queer that helped individuals become who they are today, but it can also cause a fair amount of psychological pain. For instance, many people are more familiar with LGB identities than with queer identities and have a tendency to lump queer people in with the LGB mainstream; this can be particularly erasing for queer people.

Other identities such as gender, race, class, and disability may complicate the situation because people with multiple marginalized identities are often given the message—whether implicitly or explicitly—that their differences are unacceptable or make others uncomfortable and/or anxious. Although this is often the case for all queer people, it can be especially true for queer people of color. As queer becomes more widely known as an identity in mainstream discourse, queer people of color point out that dominant queer narratives and representations of queer people are largely white, confounding feelings of alienation and erasure.

This is why the queer community and friendships with people from similar intersecting identity groups are so important to those struggling with alienation. Queer people who might feel different in similar ways can come together and support one another in their shared experiences. This, however, may be challenging for people struggling with internalized queerphobia because feelings of shame may make it difficult to connect with other queer people.

## INTERNALIZED QUEERPHOBIA

Internalized queerphobia is a common theme that comes up in therapy with queer folks. In internalized queerphobia, people may talk about their desires, feelings, and behaviors related to their queerness with disgust, self-hatred, and other self-critical appraisals. Individuals may be very active against queerphobia directed toward other people, but they may struggle to protect themselves from similar narratives directed inward.

## SHAME ABOUT SEXUALITY

For many queer patients, the ability to talk about sexuality is not a key part of psychiatric treatment. However, those for whom it is often experience shame when speaking about their sexuality. This might manifest in hypercritical thoughts or saying queerphobic things about their own desires or others in their life. It can also interact with concerns about being "queer enough" if individuals fear that their sexual behavior is heteronormative.

As with any treatment, shame can make it difficult for individuals to speak openly with a psychiatrist, so it is important not to ask too many questions about their queer sexuality and allow them to share as much as they would like to share. Additionally, some patients needing to speak about their sexuality find it helpful to work with a queer psychiatrist, although this is not true of all LGBTQ+ individuals.

## FEARS OF BEING PATHOLOGIZED

Queer people regularly worry that their psychiatrist will pathologize them or treat them in a discriminatory manner. This concern is rooted in a long history of oppression against queer people in the mental health fields, and your patient may have previously experienced discrimination by a medical professional or a mental health provider who has done one or more of the following things:

- Asked intrusive questions about the patient's sexual history and queer identity that are tangential or irrelevant to treatment
- Questioned the patient's identification as queer
- Attempted to determine the "etiology" of the patient's queerness (e.g., linking a person's queer identity to past sexual abuse—a common and offensive misconception)
- Connected the etiology of the patient's reported symptoms to their queer identity

Queer people may have also been exposed to some form of conversion therapy in an attempt to change their sexual orientation, which is not supported by any major medical or mental health organization in the United States and can have devastating impacts on the individual, including suicide.

## FEELING IMMATURE, SILLY, OR BEHIND

Because we live in a queerphobic society, queer people are often forced to disavow their queerness in certain spaces (or often altogether) during childhood, leaving them with different developmental experiences than those of heterosexual people. This can result in some queer people acknowledging or exploring their queerness later in life than heterosexual kids, who may have had the opportunity to openly explore their sexuality during adolescence. One theme that can come up in therapy with a queer person is feeling behind, silly, or immature because their experiences do not line up with heteronormative trajectories of development. At times, queer adults may express feeling adolescent or become worried that their desires are silly, immature, or inappropriate for their age.

## NAVIGATING INTERSECTING IDENTITIES AND DISCRIMINATION

As previously discussed throughout this chapter, navigating intersecting marginalized identities within (Riggs 2007) and outside the queer community can be very difficult, to say the least. For any person, queer identity carries complex connections with life experiences related to race, ethnicity, gender, class, disability status, geographical location, immigration status, and more. Intersectionality theory posits that the experiences of multiply marginalized individuals are not adequately represented by adding one type of discrimination they experience to another; rather, a person's social identities interact and intersect in ways that create a unique and more substantial experience of discrimination (Crenshaw 1989). The following two case examples show how this can play out.

### CASE EXAMPLE 3: RURAL WHITE QUEER IDENTITY

Lauren, a white, queer, cis woman (pronouns: she/her/her), is a college student from a working-class family who grew up in a rural area that she describes as "homophobic." She is currently living in a large northeastern U.S. city where, for the first time, she feels more open to exploring her queer sexuality, which she has not previously disclosed to others. As she navigates shifts related to her queer identity and her growing queer community in the city, Lauren also begins to come to terms with memories of explicit and implicit homophobia she experienced growing up that interface with her class status and white rural identity.

### CASE EXAMPLE 4: BLACK MIDWESTERN TRANS IDENTITY

Denise, a black, queer, trans woman (pronouns: she/her/her) who grew up in a middle-class suburban family, works as a lawyer in a small city in the midwestern United States. At the law firm where she works, she is read by her colleagues as a heterosexual cis woman. She is the only black person at the law firm and often experiences microaggressions by white coworkers. She is afraid of being fired if her coworkers find out she is trans, which is legal in her state.

## FAMILIAL CONFLICT AND CHOSEN FAMILIES

Because heteronormativity creates the foundation for how family is conceptualized in U.S. culture, it is common for queer people to experience conflicts with their family of origin. Many queer people experience significant queerphobia in their family of origin, through explicit or implicit language and actions of family members. Queer people often have childhood experiences of repeated invalidation, abuse, and even efforts by family members to ignore or deny their queer identity and coerce or force them to perform heterosexuality. For example, families may threaten to disown queer individuals if they engage in queer relationships or claim queer identities, forcing the individual to choose between living a queer life and having a relationship with their family.

As queer people become adults and begin to accept themselves as queer, they often have to try to come to terms with these painful familial relationships. For some people, this may mean working to be more assertive with family members to express to family members how they have been hurt or to set clearer boundaries with them. Others may need to distance themselves from their family of origin or come to terms with being cut off by their family of origin after disclosing their sexual identity. In other situations, coming out to family is neither safe nor preferable, which means learning to accept the limits of these relationships.

A common practice in the queer community is reconceptualizing kinship by creating a chosen family. For many, building a chosen queer family is central to healing from these painful family histories and can offer a loving, accepting support system.

# Conclusion

Therapists can support their queer patients by keeping in mind the many ways queer lives can differ from cisheteronormative lives, including such areas as family dynamics, sexuality, politics, discrimination, and gender identity. Some queer people are fortunate to not struggle with some of the topics discussed in this chapter, but it is helpful to be aware of these common experiences in case they arise in treatment. Many queer people enter therapeutic relationships wary of being pathologized, so keeping an open mind and maintaining awareness of your own subjectivity and social location in relation to queer identities will help the therapeutic relationship and demonstrate respect.

# FIVE TAKE-HOME POINTS

- Queer is often a politically charged identity signaling resistance to heteronormative, homonormative, and cisnormative culture. The term was reclaimed during the late 1980s and early 1990s when HIV/AIDS activists harnessed the shock value of queer's derogatory history and turned it into a powerful identity and form of political resistance. Today, queer is both an individual sexual identity used by many people and an umbrella term used to refer to the entire LGBTQ+ community.

- There is no one way to be queer. The term is flexible and resists categorization in a way that mirrors the lived experiences of people who identify as queer. Part of its flexibility lies in its gender neutrality, which makes queer popular with trans people and those who are attracted to multiple genders.

- Many people who identify as queer are marginalized within the greater LGBT community. Intersecting oppressions elevate some voices within the community—especially white, middle-class, cisgender, gay, and lesbian voices—above poor, queer, and trans people of color's voices. These compounding oppressions and erasures can also lead to different experiences of discrimination, systemic barriers, and violence.

- Psychiatry and other mental health professions have long pathologized queer identities and sexual practices, which makes some queer people hesitant to seek mental health care. Even though homosexuality was removed from DSM in 1973, these attitudes still linger in social stigma that affects queer people today. It is up to mental health providers to create a safe space for queer patients to receive the help they need.

- Providing culturally competent queer mental health care begins with education and self-reflection. Mental health providers can improve the health and well-being of the LGBTQ+ community and increase access to queer-friendly psychotherapy and psychiatric services by educating themselves and by challenging antiquated notions of human sexuality. Reflecting on one's own experience can help providers use what they have learned in order to provide patient-centered care while keeping any personal anxieties or nonclinically relevant curiosities at bay.

# Resources

Association of LGBTQ Psychiatrists, www.aglp.org
Division 44: Society for the Psychology of Sexual Orientation and Gender Diversity, American Psychological Association, www.apadivisions.org/division-44
GLBT Historical Society, www.glbthistory.org
National Alliance on Mental Illness: LGBTQ, www.nami.org/find-support/lgbtq
them. (news, culture, and current events coverage for the LGBTQ+ community), www.them.us

# References

American Psychiatric Association: Sexual deviation, in Diagnostic and Statistical Manual: Mental Disorders. Washington, DC, American Psychiatric Association, 1952, pp 38–39
American Psychiatric Association: Diagnostic and Statistical Manual of Mental Disorders, 2nd Edition. Washington, DC, American Psychiatric Association, 1968
American Psychiatric Association: Diagnostic and Statistical Manual of Mental Disorders, 3rd Edition. Washington, DC, American Psychiatric Association, 1980
Burnes TR, Singh AA, Witherspoon RG: Sex positivity and counseling psychology: an introduction to the major contribution. Couns Psychol 45(4):470–486, 2017
Burnes TR, Stanley JL (eds): Teaching LGBTQ Psychology: Queering Innovative Pedagogy and Practice. Washington, DC, American Psychological Association, 2017

Butler J: Doing justice to someone: sex reassignment and allegories of transsexuality, in Undoing Gender. New York, Routledge, 2004a, pp 57–74

Butler J: Undoing Gender. New York, Routledge, 2004b

Cava P: Activism, politics, and organizing, in Trans Bodies, Trans Selves: A Resource for the Transgender Community. Edited by Erickson-Schroth L. New York, Oxford University Press, 2014, pp 567–589

Combahee River Collective: The Combahee River Collective statement (1977), in Home Girls: A Black Feminist Anthology, 2nd Edition. Edited by Smith B. New Brunswick, NJ, Rutgers University Press, 2000, pp 264–274

Crenshaw K: Demarginalizing the intersection of race and sex: a black feminist critique of antidiscrimination doctrine, feminist theory and antiracist politics. University of Chicago Legal Forum 140:139–167, 1989

Duggan L: The Twilight of Equality? Neoliberalism, Cultural Politics, and the Attack on Democracy. Boston, MA, Beacon Press, 2003

Hardy JW, Easton D: The Ethical Slut: A Practical Guide to Polyamory, Open Relationships, and Other Freedoms in Sex and Love, 3rd Edition. Berkeley, CA, Ten Speed Press, 2017

James SE, Herman JL, Rankin S, et al: The Report of the 2015 U.S. Transgender Survey. Washington, DC, National Center for Transgender Equality, 2016

Kelly RC: Introduction to queer theory, in Trans Bodies, Trans Selves: A Resource for the Transgender Co mmunity. Edited by Erickson-Schroth L. New York, Oxford University Press, 2014, pp 82–83

Kolmes K, Stock W, Moser C: Investigating bias in psychotherapy with BDSM clients. J Homosex 50(2–3):301–324, 2006 16803769

Levounis P, Anson AJ: Sexual identity in patient-therapist relationships, in The LGBT Casebook. Edited by Levounis P, Drescher J, Barber ME. Washington, DC, American Psychiatric Publishing, 2012, pp 73–83

Moradi B: (Re)focusing intersectionality: from social identities back to systems of oppression and privilege, in Handbook of Sexual Orientation and Gender Diversity in Counseling and Psychotherapy. Edited by DeBord KA, Fischer AR, Bieschke KJ, et al. Washington, DC, American Psychological Association, 2017, pp 105–127

Ortmann DM, Sprott RA: Sexual Outsiders: Understanding BDSM Sexualities and Communities. Lanham, MD, Rowman and Littlefield, 2013

Platt LF, Wolf JK, Scheitle CP: Patterns of mental health care utilization among sexual orientation minority groups. J Homosex 65(2):135–153, 2018 28346079

Riggs D: Queer theory and its future in psychology: exploring issues of race privilege. Soc Pers Psychol Compass 1(1):39–52, 2007

Shilts R: And the band played on: Politics, people, and the AIDS epidemic (1987), eBook Edition. London, Souvenir Press, 2011

Sprott RA, Benoit Hadcock B: Bisexuality, pansexuality, queer identity, and kink identity. Sex Relation Ther 33(1–2):214–232, 2018

Stryker S: Transgender History: The Roots of Today's Revolution, 2nd Edition. Berkeley, CA, Seal Press, 2017

Taormino T: Opening Up: A Guide to Creating and Sustaining Open Relationships. San Francisco, CA, Cleis Press, 2008

Taormino T (ed): The Ultimate Guide to Kink: BDSM, Role Play and the Erotic Edge. Berkeley, CA, Cleis Press, 2012

Vaid-Menon A: Queer impossibility. ALOK (website), November 29, 2018. Available at: www.alokvmenon.com/blog/2018/11/29/queer-impossibility. Accessed February 2, 2020.

# Chapter 6

# Questioning

## The Second Q in LGBTQ$^2$IAPA

MARK JOSEPH MESSIH, M.D., M.SC.

The power to question is the basis of all human progress.

*Indira Gandhi*

## Psychological and Cultural Context

How do we define what it means to be "questioning?" How is sexual identity developed, and how has that process changed in the twenty-first century? How does the term *questioning* compare with such terms as *bisexual* or *fluid*? Talking about questioning means talking, briefly, about sexual development, cultural studies on sexuality, and identity. With that in mind, the goal of the following subsection is to give a general, informative overview of a very large field of study to help clinicians working with people who are questioning their sexuality.

In this chapter, we look at the concept of questioning through different lenses to help providers understand patients' experiences and provide informed care. First, what does it mean to be questioning? Second, what are the common concerns that patients, parents, and physicians have? Finally, what are the common concerns that arise during treatment, and how can providers address them?

### WHAT IS "QUESTIONING?" AN EVOLVING CONCEPT

Our understanding of questioning sexuality has evolved dramatically over the nineteenth and twentieth centuries. One way to think about the change in our knowledge is to imagine that sexuality used to be seen as a set of steps from homosexual to heterosexual. Questioning was part of a process to figure out a default heterosexual identity. In other words, psychological explanations of navigating sexuality saw questioning as a linear process, with people going through a series of steps to realize their "true" sexual identity. Over time, this process became less of a set of steps and more of a Venn diagram, with different pieces of someone's sense of self overlapping to make up their sexuality.

## FREUD'S THOUGHTS ON QUESTIONING SEXUALITY

Freud's psychosexual developmental theory is an example of a linear model (de Kuyper 1993). If a patient failed to move through a set of subsequent stages, this, and overidentification with the mother, would result in the patient's becoming homosexual. Therapy focused on helping patients discover their heterosexual identity and labeled homosexuality as a disorder. Freud explored any of these ideas around 1905 and published them in one his most famous works, *Three Essays on the Theory of Sexuality* (Freud 1949).

## ENTER THE MATRIX: THE NEXT GENERATION OF QUESTIONING THEORY

After Freud, research went in a different direction. In the 1950s and 1960s, researchers developed scales and matrixes in which homosexuality was not necessarily the opposite of heterosexuality or a pathological state but a different identity on a spectrum of possible orientations. One famous example is the Kinsey scale (Figure 6–1), which placed sexual orientation on a 0–6 scale from exclusively homosexual to exclusively heterosexual.

Over the course of the twentieth and twenty-first centuries, theories of sexuality have become more nuanced, separating out considerations such as sexual practices, identity, and attraction into distinct facets of identity. In 1985, Fredrich Klein devised the Klein Sexual Orientation Grid (Klein 1985, 1993), which expanded on Kinsey's concepts but introduced new dimensions into the mix. First, Klein asked patients to rate experiences over different time frames: past, present, and ideal (what they would choose in the future if possible). Then, patients were asked about multiple areas of their sexuality, including behaviors, fantasies, and self-identification.

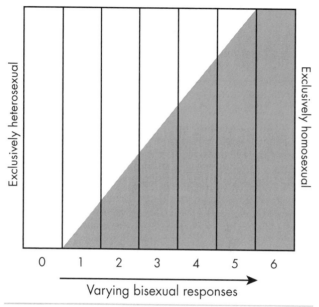

Exclusively heterosexual

Exclusively homosexual

0    1    2    3    4    5    6

Varying bisexual responses

FIGURE 6–1.  **Kinsey scale.**

## QUESTIONING SEXUALITY AND HOW PATIENTS SEE THEMSELVES

In 1979, Vivienne Cass introduced the Homosexual Identity Formation (HIF) stage model (Cass 1979; Halpin and Allen 2004), which looked at the relationships between people and their social environment. She argued that someone's sexual identity is related to three considerations:

1. How do people see themselves?
2. What are their sexual behaviors?
3. How do they think other people see them?

Questioning sexuality was becoming less about preferences in the bedroom and more about how people see themselves, how they understand being straight or gay, and how their community sees being straight or gay. Dr. Cass put forward a set of steps that people go through as they question their sexuality:

1. Identity confusion
2. Identity comparison

*Questioning*                                                      **111**

3. Identity tolerance
4. Identity acceptance
5. Identity pride
6. Identity synthesis

There is one concern raised by this theory that we should keep in mind as providers. Some people look at the HIF model and see it as a setup of steps (similar to Freud's theory) that assume people are either heterosexual or homosexual, and if someone has not moved through all these stages, they have not figured out whether they are homosexual or heterosexual. Halpin and Allen (2004) raise this point because it resonates with a reported experience patients have when talking about their questioning to others. Sometimes people—both heterosexual and homosexual—may try to tell someone who is questioning to "just" come out or rush them to "figure it out." It is harmful to assume that questioning people have not come out or accepted themselves because this can have the opposite of the intended effect, isolating a questioning person from both LGBTQ+ and heterosexual communities. The takeaway point is that you should not assume that a patient's questioning of their sexuality is a pathology in and of itself. Instead, questioning is an ongoing process with many factors that should be considered.

## A DEFINITION OF QUESTIONING

Questioning can be defined as ongoing developmental experience that brings together the patient's feelings, drives, desires, sense of self, biology, and relationship history. With this idea in mind, in the next subsection, we explore the main areas of research with regard to questioning sexuality to help clinicians become aware of issued to keep in mind when working with different patient groups. Areas of research include the variations in questioning between men and women and between races and by age.

## RESEARCH

How do people from different communities come to understand their sexual identity? Katz-Wise et al. (2017) focused on the differences in how men and women process their sexuality and came up with a list of milestones, or important life experiences, and time frames for when they happen in a person's life. These experiences include same-gender attrac-

**TABLE 6–1.** Milestones in processing sexuality

| Milestone | Age in years at which milestone is reached | |
| --- | --- | --- |
| | **Females** | **Males** |
| Same-gender attraction | 17 | 15 |
| Other-gender attraction | 10 | 10 |
| Same-gender sexual experience | 18 | 15 |
| Other-gender sexual experience | 16 | 17 |
| Sexual minority identity | 17–18 | 16–17 |

*Source.*   Katz-Wise et al. 2017.

tion, other-gender attraction, same-gender sexual experience, other-gender sexual experience, and sexual identity formation. As outlined in Table 6–1, men reach these milestones at younger ages compared with women in heterosexual, bisexual, and homosexual categories (Katz-Wise et al. 2017). There are two takeaway point from this work. First, the process of questioning one's sexuality has multiple dimensions. Second, it can be helpful to frame discussion of sexual questioning by looking at experiences, desires, and identity development.

Researchers are also exploring how the experience of questioning sexuality can differ by race. Experiences of racism within the LGBT community and homophobia from one's racial community can make it difficult to question and disclose sexual identity (Parks et al. 2004). In addition, questioning identity is informed by both the local environment and broader social norms. How do culture and identity shape the ways patients understand sexuality? Are sexual minorities stigmatized within their racial community?

Recently, questioning sexuality has become a topic of the general public's social experience. More and more, online resources, support groups in schools, television programs, and social media are showing characters who are navigating their sexual identity. Consequently, the languages of identity and questioning are changing. The visibility of communities of bisexual, asexual, and polyamorous individuals in mainstream television shows helps youth find representations of themselves that make it easier to talk about sexuality if they are in a safe space to do so (Darwish 2018; Novick 2017; Viera 2019).

For teenagers, sexual attraction, romantic attraction, and overall identity can differ from one another (Savin-Williams 2015). Some teenagers see labels as unrelatable and inappropriate for an attraction to a specific person or people. Others may have difficulty with questioning identity out of fear of consequences of what it means to identify as gay.

## Questions Well-Meaning People Ask

**Lesbian, gay, bisexual, bicurious, queer—how do people figure out where they fit in?**

Sexual orientation is a big part of a person's identity, involving physical attraction, emotional connection, and other parts of identity. It takes time to sort through feelings as they develop, and it is a normal and healthy part of everyone's development to go through such questioning. One way to navigate this journey is for the questioning individual to talk with people they trust and with whom they feel safe. Some people have supportive individuals in their life they can talk to, such as parents, close friends, physicians, school staff, spiritual advisors, or online support. For additional sources of support, see the list of resources at the end of this chapter. When discussing a patient's experiences, it is often useful to provide descriptions of different communities (Green 2015). Table 6–2 provides descriptions of complex identities; these definitions are very succinct but can be helpful in navigating the process of sexual identity with patients.

For many people, it takes time to figure out their feelings. Some people know from an early age; others discover feelings later in life. Many people start thinking about their sexuality as teenagers, but many others do so as adults, so there is no rush to "figure it out." It is also important to keep in mind that sexual orientation is more than sexual activity; it also includes romantic love, physical attraction, and community. Some people benefit from looking up descriptions of different communities, which helps sort their experiences (see resources at the end of the chapter).

**TABLE 6–2.** Terminology for sexual identity and sexual attraction

| Term | Definition |
|------|-----------|
| Asexual | Not sexually attracted to anyone or does not have a sexual orientation |
| Bicurious | Curiosity about having sexual relations with a person of the same gender or sex |
| Bigender | Gender identity that is a combination of male and female |
| Bisexual | Emotional, physical, and/or sexual attraction to males and females |
| Gay | Male-identified individuals who are attracted to males in a romantic, erotic, and/or emotional sense |
| Genderqueer | A gender-variant person whose identity is neither male nor female; this can mean identity is beyond gender or a combination of genders |
| Intergender | Gender identity between genders or a combination of genders |
| Lesbian | Female-identified individuals who are attracted to females in a romantic, erotic, and/or emotional sense |
| Queer | A matrix of sexual preferences, orientations, and habits of people who are not exclusively heterosexual and/or monogamous; includes lesbians, gay men, bisexuals, and trans people |
| Transgender | Individuals whose gender expression and/or identity differs from conventional expectations based on the sex they were born into |

*Source.* Green 2015.

**How can someone know their sexual orientation if they are not having sex?**

Having sex is only one part of figuring out sexual identity. Most adolescents will have crushes when they are young, before they have sex. Thinking about emotions, feelings, and attraction is another way of approaching this question. Also, different people start to experience sexual attraction at different ages. It is not a requirement to be sexually active to identify with a specific orientation.

**Is there something wrong with me?**

Absolutely not! Questioning your sexuality is completely normal. Multiple medical groups, including the American Psychiatric Association, the American Psychological Association, and the American Medical Association, all agree that LGBTQ+ identities are not a disease. However, although being LGBTQ+ is certainly not a disease, some people have to deal with hardships because of their identity. These hardships are responses to the stress and stigma many LGBTQ+ people face, and sometimes they increase the risk of anxiety, depression, or substance use. If you experience such feelings, it is not because questioning is wrong.

**I assumed LGBT people look or act a certain way. What if I don't fit in. Am I still part of the community?**

There are many ways of acting within LGBTQ+ communities, just as within heterosexual groups. Certain stereotypes of a community often get more attention through media, but they are only a fraction of a big community. Stereotypes often come from not knowing more about a group of people, so one way to learn about different ways of being is to read up on cultural figures and reach out to a local community group for information. One resource is the website for LGBT History Month (www.lgbthistorymonth.com), a database that provides information on a diverse range of people and their contributions to LGBT communities.

**Are there health implications associated with questioning identity?**

A lot of researchers have looked at health outcomes within LGBT populations; however, not much has been reported on questioning youth (Shearer et al. 2016). Although studies suggest that compared with heterosexual and LGBT people, questioning youth are more likely to be bullied and experience adverse mental health outcomes such as anxiety, depression, and suicidal thoughts, there are a lot of contextual factors to acknowledge (Birkett et al. 2009). Questioning is impacted by the environment a person is in. Do they have people to ask questions of? Are there examples of people with different sexual identities in their lives? What does their cultural community think of different sexual identities? Thus, although there is no direct health implication from questioning identity, there are contextual factors at work that can make the process difficult and, unfortunately, at times unsafe. It is helpful for parents, teachers, and clinicians to tell someone who questions their sexuality that they are not sick.

### My child is questioning their sexuality and is asking for support. What should I do?

Many parents feel anxious talking about sexuality and are unsure about how to handle it. Most adults did not have conversations like that with their own parents, so it is a tough talk to have. Some parents ask if questioning sexuality means that the parent did something wrong. First, there is nothing wrong with your child. Second, no, you did not do anything wrong. Parents may have negative stereotypes of the LGBTQ+ community and may worry about their children's health. One way of navigating these concerns is to reach out to other parents in the community or online about their experiences.

More research is being done to determine an ideal time for talking about sexuality with adolescents, but it is important to note that talking about sex with teenagers does not prompt them to start becoming sexually active or change their sexuality (Flores and Barroso 2017). Conversations about sexuality are often reactive and happen once pubertal changes become visible. Teenagers may find such conversations awkward and intrusive. Adolescents questioning their sexuality prefer reciprocal discussions instead of a lecture format. Also, some parents expect children to initiate the conversation when the child has questions, whereas children might expect their parents to start the conversation. If parents and kids have different ideas on who should start a conversation, this can lead to the whole conversation being avoided all together. In general, it is better, when possible, for parents to make the first step, saying that they are here to talk when their child is ready.

**I am a pediatrician working with teenagers. How can I better serve LGBTQ+ teens?**

Several guidelines have been put forward by the American Association of Pediatricians on working with LGBTQ+ communities (Committee on Adolescence 2013). Structural changes that physicians can make include making forms and questions gender neutral (e.g., asking if a female patient is in a relationship versus asking if they have a boyfriend). It is a good idea for you to use neutral terms so the patient does not think that you are biased either way. If teenagers do not feel comfortable talking about their sexuality, they might use gender-neutral terms to talk about crushes or relationships. For example, if a clinician asks how a male patient's girlfriend is doing, the patient may respond by saying "they're fine" as opposed to saying "he is fine" or correcting the provider.

Although higher rates of depression and substance use are reported in sexual minority and questioning youth (Shearer et al. 2016), you should reassure patients (and their parents) that being part of this group is not abnormal or a cause of mental illness—rather, such problems are often caused by homophobia. Some LGBTQ+ youth who come to you for treatment may have had negative health care interactions in the past, which can make it difficult for them to bring up health concerns. Be upfront. Let the patient know you are an LGBTQ+ supportive provider through items on the walls, decorative pins, or other symbols patients see when they come to your office. Use terms that the patient uses, such as *gay* instead of *homosexual*.

**I am a psychotherapist. Do you have any tips for working with questioning patients?**

Questioning patients may come into therapy to get support for stress related to their sexual identity. Other times, support for the patient's questioning might not be a treatment goal to start with even if the therapist thinks it should be a priority. Stressors specific to LGBTQ+ life include homophobia, heterosexism, and internalized homophobia. Homophobia refers to fear, hatred, discomfort with, or mistrust of people who are lesbian, gay, or bisexual. Heterosexism refers to social norms that stigmatize nonheterosexual behaviors, identities, relationships, or communities. Internalized homophobia refers to LGBTQ+ people taking in negative representations of nonheterosexuality.

The minority stress model is a framework that looks at the connections between someone's sexual identity and the stressors to which they are exposed and how those connections impact health (Meyer and Frost 2013). Being part of a sexual minority is linked to being a victim of discrimination and violence (Kozuch 2019). Patients may also talk about the stress of expecting to be rejected and of actual rejection. Other stressors include the anxiety of hiding their identity from people in their lives and self-hatred because of their questioning.

Sometimes, therapists bring their own preconceptions into treatment. For example, a therapist may assume that LGBTQ+ patients, especially gay men, are less able to commit to relationships. Therapists may believe that bisexuality is just a phase or consider questioning people to be less "stable" in some way than other sexual minorities. All of these preconceptions can be damaging to the patient-therapist relationship and can hinder treatment; therapists should avoid bringing such preconceptions into therapy.

Therapists at times feel pressured to push patients into making decisions and coming out prematurely, which may be more damaging than healing to someone who is not ready to assume a sexual orientation identity. External factors, such as risk of violence or social ostracism, may account for people's reluctance come out (Association of Gay and Lesbian Psychiatrists 2012). Strategies for making the patient comfortable even before entering treatment include use of forms, staff training, and use of appropriate language (Gay and Lesbian Medical Association 2006). Patients may feel at ease finding providers through referral programs, including LGBTQ+ organizations or through advertisements in LGBTQ+ media. Small changes to intake forms, such as changing "marital status" to "relationship status" are recommended. Providers can consider adding transgender to the male/female check boxes on intake forms. During the interview, it is recommended that providers use gender-neutral language (e.g., "partner" or "significant others"), ask open-ended questions, and avoid assumptions about the gender of a patient's sexual partners. For more information on working with LGBTQ+ patients, see the Resources section.

## Themes that May Emerge in Therapy

Learning that a patient is questioning their sexuality can happen at any time over the course of therapy. In some cases, questioning is the main reason someone comes for treatment, whereas with other patients, it could come up much later in therapy. There are several tips for navigating the history taking and initial conversations around questioning (Heggestad and Wetsch 2010). For example, clinicians can acknowledge how brave the patient is in sharing that they are questioning their sexuality. The clinician should also normalize the patient's questioning.

Themes to consider during therapy include the following:

- Safety assessments and confidentiality
- Assessing the patient's understanding of sexuality
- Exploring connections between race and sexuality
- Questioning as an older adult

## RISKS OF HARM WHEN QUESTIONING SEXUALITY

Teenagers may be at risk of harm or being kicked out of their home. Approximately 40% of homeless youth identify as LGBT (National Coalition for the Homeless 2018); these youth felt unsafe after coming out or were forced out of their homes by family members. To determine the risks of harm at home, therapists can ask patients how they think their family might respond to their questioning. Have family members made comments that suggest they would be supportive? Have they made comments that suggest they would be against their child being anything other than heterosexual? Does the family follow any cultural norms that might indicate whether family members would be supportive or discouraging of questioning?

If the patient reports a significant amount of distress related to understanding their sexuality and the family seems supportive, consider including family members in treatment. As part of helping families to accept a child's identity, researchers have recommended an approach that encompasses the following: exposing myths, reviewing impact of family reactions on LGBTQ+ youth, discussing conflict and rejection, and validating the family's uncertainty and concerns (Ryan 2009). Myths include the belief that only adults can know their sexuality or the belief that being LGBTQ+ is temporary. Discuss how the family's response affects the patient. If conflict and rejection are present, youth are more likely to experience adverse health outcomes, including elevated levels of depression and increased rates of suicide attempts, illicit substance use, and anxiety. Parents who are concerned or uncertain about how to proceed may report loving their child but not knowing how to support them. Ways of supporting a child can include talking to them about their LGBTQ+ identity, expressing affection when told their child is LGBTQ+, supporting them even when feeling uncomfortable, and believing your child can have a happy future as an LGBTQ+ adult. For additional strategies, see the Resources section.

## PATIENT'S UNDERSTANDING OF SEXUALITY

When working a patient who is questioning their sexuality, ask the patient about their own understanding of sexuality. Is it a physical connection, an emotional connection, and/or a lifestyle they identify with? It can be helpful for the patient to learn that sexuality has components of each, and they can reflect on which of these components aligns better with their feelings about their sexuality. Another question to consider is how the patient's understanding of sexuality is impacted by race.

## RACE AND QUESTIONING SEXUALITY

Studies show that some racial groups experience homophobia more frequently than others, particularly from members of their own community. Daboin et al. (2015), for example, found higher rates of homophobia among blacks than whites. In addition, racialization, which refers to the different ways in which a society construct races as real, different, and unequal in ways that impact an individual's economic, political, and social life, can contribute to internalized homophobia. In working through issues related to race, it may be helpful to raise the following questions:

- Did the patient grow up in a conservative religious environment?
- Was there a lack of visible sexual minorities in the patient's community?
- What messages about questioning sexuality has the patient internalized from society and how are they processing those messages?

Different communities report questioning sexuality at different ages. One study of adult women who identified as lesbians found differences in the age of questioning sexuality, deciding sexuality, and disclosing identity to family and relationships between minority and white women (Parks et al.

2004). This study suggested that African American and Latinx women questioned their sexuality earlier (14.4 and 14.5 years, respectively) than white women (17.5 years). The study also looked at time between questioning sexuality and disclosing lesbian status to family members and found a shorter period of time for white women than for African American and Latinx women. This could be due to the increased visibility and acceptance of white lesbians in comparison to minority populations.

Research with minority questioning male patients suggests that questioning happens at the same time that individuals are figuring out their cultural and ethnic identity (Jamil et al. 2009). In their research, Jamil et al. discussed the idea of ethnic identity formation by turning to community resources, family members, peers, and cultural practices. In contrast, sexual identity development was seen as more private and solitary, with participants seeking out organizations specifically catering to LGBTQ+ youth. They further went on to note the presence of "contrasting experiences of oppression" such as experiencing racism from the broader heterosexual community and objectification by the LGBTQ+ community due to their ethnicity. This is not to say that people from certain groups will necessarily have more resistance to questioning sexuality or face more challenges in their journey. Being mindful of context and being open to learning from the patient about their environment is a valuable component of understanding the patient better.

## QUESTIONING AND OLDER ADULTS

Another issue that can emerge during therapy is the age of patients when they are questioning their sexuality. Approximately 2.7 million individuals older than age 50 identify as LGBT, and knowledge about sexual questioning and identity in this group is limited (Jamil et al. 2009). However, researchers have examined how the era in which individuals were born and the environment in which they grew up shaped the process of questioning their sexuality (Fredriksen-Goldsen and Kim 2017). Patients who started exploring their sexuality during the 1950s and 1960s were exposed to anti-gay messages and the classification of homosexuality as a mental disorder. This group is referred to as the Silenced Generation. This group was followed by the Pride Generation, which refers to people who came of age during a time of sweeping changes in social norms. These changes include the sexual revolution, the Stonewall riots, the women's movement, and removal of homosexuality from DSM in 1973 (American Psychiatric Association 1973). There will be variation within age groups depending on the patient's social, economic, and racial context, but patients' age can impact how they understand, express, and accept sexual questioning.

## Conclusion

The question of sexuality is a core part of a person's identity. It connects with desires, romantic love, self-image, and self-expression. Our understanding of questioning sexuality has changed over the past century, which reflects how complex this experience is. Each patient's journey is shaped by many internal considerations and external forces. Internal factors include what an individual understands sexuality to mean and the person's inner sense of positive or negative ideas around sexuality. Different communities privilege heterosexuality above other identities, and in certain contexts, homosexuality is devalued and even criminalized. The messages individuals receive from peers, the media, role models, and family members shape how their questioning takes place.

Working with questioning patients gives clinicians an incredible opportunity to bear witness to a critical part of a person's development and help them discover fascinating parts of their identity. The process of reflecting on one's sexuality is not pathological and does not predispose someone to mental illness. Rather, the emotional distress associated with questioning comes from perceived consequences, loss of family and friends, and social isolation. Questioning individuals benefit from supportive, nonjudgmental friends and family, and patients should be referred to appropriate community resources to help them build new relationships.

## FIVE TAKE-HOME POINTS

- Questioning sexuality is a normal, healthy part of development.
- Questioning youth are at increased risk of stigmatization, violence, and internalized homophobia.

- Sexuality is understood and experienced differently by each individual and is shaped by biological forces, cultural norms, and race.
- Create a supportive, nonjudgmental environment to promote conversations with patients about sexuality.
- Connect the patient to appropriate community resources where they can learn more about different sexual identities and see what is right for them.

## Resources

American Academy of Pediatrics: Gay, lesbian, and bisexual teens: facts for teens and their parents. The AAP Parenting Website, www.healthychildren.org/English/ages-stages/teen/dating-sex/Pages/Gay-Lesbian-and-Bisexual-Teens-Facts-for-Teens-and-Their-Parents.aspx

Fenway Health Data Collection Toolkit, https://doaskdotell.org

Fenway Institute, https://fenwayhealth.org/the-fenway-institute

It Gets Better Project, https://itgetsbetter.org

National LGBTQ Task Force, www.thetaskforce.org

The Trevor Project, www.thetrevorproject.org

## References

American Psychiatric Association: Homosexuality and sexual orientation disturbance: proposed change in DSM-II, 6th printing, page 44. APA Document Ref No 730008. Washington, DC, American Psychiatric Association, 1973. Available at: https://dsm.psychiatry online.org/doi/pdf/10.1176/appi.books.9780890420362.dsm-ii-6thprintingchange. Accessed: November 25, 2019.

Association of Gay and Lesbian Psychiatrists: General issues in working with GLBT patients, in LGBT Mental Health Syllabus. Philadelphia, PA, Association of Gay and Lesbian Psychiatrists, 2012. Available at: www.aglp.org/gap/4_psychotherapy/#general. Accessed November 10, 2019.

Birkett M, Espelage DL, Koenig B: LGB and questioning students in schools: the moderating effects of homophobic bullying and school climate on negative outcomes. J Youth Adolesc 38(7):989–1000, 2009 19636741

Bruggman A, Ortiz-Hartman K (eds): Lesbian, gay, bisexual, transgender, and questioning youth: psychosocial issues, in Salem Health: Community and Family Health Issues, Vol 2 (E–M). Amenia, NY, Grey House Publishing, 2017, pp 1018–1022

Cass VC: Homosexual identity formation: a theoretical model. J Homosex 4(3):219–235, 1979 264126

Committee on Adolescence: Office-based care for lesbian, gay, bisexual, transgender, and questioning youth. Pediatrics 132(1):198–203, 2013 23796746

Daboin I, Peterson JL, Parrott DJ: Racial differences in sexual prejudice and its correlates among heterosexual men. Cultur Divers Ethnic Minor Psychol 21(2):258–267, 2015 25602467

Darwish M: 6 asexual characters that have changed TV. New York, TV Insider, April 2, 2018. Available at: www.tvinsider.com/gallery/asexual-characters-on-tv. Accessed February 1, 2020.

de Kuyper E: The Freudian construction of sexuality: the gay foundations of heterosexuality and straight homophobia. J Homosex 24(3–4):137–144, 1993 8505533

Flores D, Barroso J: 21st century parent-child sex communication in the U.S.: a process review. OpenAIRE, 2017. Available at: www.open aire.eu/search/publication?articleId=od_____267::fbe01505391 a983f5359379b5423f467. Accessed November 8, 2019.

Fredriksen-Goldsen K, Kim H: The science of conducting research with LGBT older adults—an introduction to aging with pride: National Health, Aging, and Sexuality/Gender study (NHAS). Gerontologist 57(suppl 1):S1–S14, 2017 28087791

Freud S: Three essays on the Theory of Sexuality. London, Imago, 1949

Gay and Lesbian Medical Association: Guidelines for care of lesbian, gay, bisexual, and transgender patients. Washington, DC, Gay and Lesbian Medical Association, 2006. Available at: www.rainbow welcome.org/uploads/pdfs/GLMA%20guidelines%202006%20 FINAL.pdf. Accessed on February 10, 2020.

Green EI: LGBTQI Terminology. Los Angeles, LGBT Resource Center, University of Southern California, May 2015. Available at: https://lgbtrc.usc.edu/files/2015/05/LGBT-Terminology.pdf. Accessed February 1, 2020.

Halpin SA, Allen MW: Changes in psychosocial well-being during stages of gay identity development. J Homosex 47(2):109–126, 2004 15271626

Heggestad K, Wetsch P: Counseling gay and questioning minors about coming out. Virtual Mentor 12(8):654–657, 2010 23186851

Jamil OB, Harper GW, Fernandez MI: Sexual and ethnic identity development among gay-bisexual-questioning (GBQ) male ethnic minority adolescents. Cultur Divers Ethnic Minor Psychol 15(3):203–214, 2009 19594249

Katz-Wise SL, Rosario M, Calzo JP, et al: Endorsement and timing of sexual orientation developmental milestones among sexual minority young adults in the Growing Up Today Study. J Sex Res 54(2):172–185, 2017 27148762

Klein F, Sepekoff B, Wolf TJ: Sexual orientation: a multi-variable dynamic process. J Homosex 11(1–2):35–49, 1985 4056393

Klein F: The Bisexual Option, 2nd Edition. New York, Haworth Press, 1993

Kozuch E: HRC responds to new FBI report showing spike in reported hate crimes targeting LGBTQ people. Washington, DC, Human Rights Campaign, November 12, 2019. Available at: www.hrc.org/blog/hrc-responds-to-new-fbi-report-showing-spike-in-reported-hate-crimes-target. Accessed February 10, 2020.

Meyer IH, Frost DM: Minority stress and the health of sexual minorities, in Handbook of Psychology and Sexual Orientation. Edited by Patterson CJ, D'Augelli AR. New York, Oxford University Press, 2013, pp 252–266

National Coalition for the Homeless: LGBT Homelessness. Washington, DC, National Coalition for the Homeless, 2018. Available at: https://nationalhomeless.org/issues/lgbt. Accessed January 8, 2019.

Novick I: TV is finally starting to get polyamory right. New York, Vice, April 10, 2017. Available at: www.vice.com/en_us/article/vvk5q9/tv-is-finally-starting-to-get-polyamory-right. Accessed February 1, 2020.

Parks C, Hughes T, Matthews A: Race/ethnicity and sexual orientation: intersecting identities. Cultur Divers Ethnic Minor Psychol 10(3):241–254, 2004 15311977

Ryan C: Supportive families, healthy children: helping families with lesbian, gay, bisexual & transgender children. San Francisco, CA: Family Acceptance Project, Marian Wright Edelman Institute, San Francisco State University, 2009

Savin-Williams RC: Why the new gay teenager?, in The New Gay Teenager. Cambridge, MA, Harvard University Press, 2015, pp 1–22

Shearer A, Herres J, Kodish T, et al: Differences in mental health symptoms across lesbian, gay, bisexual, and questioning youth in primary care settings. J Adolesc Health 59(1):38–43, 2016 27053400

Viera M: Bisexuality is fluid, and TV is finally catching up. New York, Vibe, July 15, 2019. Available at: www.vibe.com/photos/bisexuality-tv-representation. Accessed February 1, 2020.

# Chapter 7

# Intersex

## *The I in LGBTQ²IAPA*

ADRIAN JACQUES H. AMBROSE, M.D.,
M.P.H., FAPA

A rose by any other name would smell as sweet.

*William Shakespeare, Romeo and Juliet, Act II, Scene II*

## Psychological and Cultural Context

Traditionally, the term *intersex* has been used most often to characterize abnormal virilization of external genitalia, which generally signifies pathologies in hormonal synthesis or effect (e.g., hyperandrogen synthesis in congenital adrenal hyperplasia, androgen receptor defects in androgen insensitivity syndrome). On the other hand, the term *disorder of sex development* (DSD) is an all-encompassing terminology for atypical presentations and/or development of genitalia, chromosomes, gonads, and hormones. In the past, common names for intersex individuals with DSD included hermaphrodite, pseudomale/pseudofemale, undermasculinized male, virilized female, and sex reversal. For many patients, this archaic nomenclature is considered to be offensive and pejorative. As a result, in this chapter we will generally use DSD as an umbrella term for this clinical condition; the term intersex is generally avoided because of its medical and nosological imprecision. At the same time, cultural sensitivity leads us to acknowledge that some people in the community prefer the term "intersex" as a form of reclaiming identity empowerment. As a result, we strongly encourage asking individuals directly for their preferred nomenclature.

The clinical approach to and understanding of the DSD population have undergone several significant transformations within the past century. However, it is especially important to note potential controversies surrounding the "disorder" part of DSD, which may be stigmatizing for a vulnerable minority population that has been historically pathologized by the medical community. As a result, some communities may refer to DSD as a condition of *differences of sex development*. This topic will be discussed further in the next subsection.

## HISTORY

For patients with ambiguous genitalia, gender assignment was often contingent on the gender binary. In addition, the process of surgically assigning a gender was based primarily on determining the "true sex" from the predominant appearance of the patient's external genitalia. Toward the end of the nineteenth century, the sex assignment process relied on gonads and histology and, subsequently, with the technological advances of the twentieth century, chromosomal testing—the center of the true sex policy (Meyer-Bahlburg 1999).

Around the 1950s, a group of Johns Hopkins clinicians and researchers reviewed the existing literature of the population with DSD and concluded that sex assigned at birth will almost always persist into adulthood, regardless of the biological sex basis (Money et al. 1955). In other words, the Hopkins group suggested that gender rearing, or nurture, had a much larger impact than biological sex, or nature. Therefore, they proposed an optimal gender policy, in which clinicians should strive to identify the "optimal" gender for a patient in terms of sexuality, psychological development, and reproductive potentials (Meyer-Bahlburg 1999, 2015). One of the researchers, John Money, touted a longitudinal case study, "The John/Joan Case," as evidence for the social learning theory of gender identity. The case examined a pair of identical twin boys, one of whom received genital reconstruction surgery and exogenous hormones, and how the gender reassignment treatments affected their early postnatal sexual differentiation. The authors of the case study concluded, erroneously, that social influences early in life could predict and shape psychosexual developments in children. There was a strong emphasis on early evaluation, often perinatally if possible, and surgical interventions to assign/reassign genders for patients. Furthermore, the optimal gender policy recommended early constructions of gender-congruent genitalia in order to "optimize" subsequent gender-congruent upbringing and psychosexual development. Replacing the true sex policy, the optimal gender policy was the principal guideline for clinical care of most individuals with DSD well into the late twentieth century.

Around 2006, an interdisciplinary group of international experts on individuals with DSD published a consensus statement that reviewed existing evidence on clinical care and outcomes of DSDs. Endorsed by the Lawson Wilkins Pediatric Endocrine Society and European Society for Paediatric Endocrinology, the consensus statement, subsequently known as the Chicago Consensus, also proposed a unifying nomenclature—disorder of sex development—to encompass congenital conditions of atypical development in gonads, chromosomes, and sex anatomies (Hughes et al. 2006). The clinical guidelines deemphasized the role of surgical interventions in cosmetic appearance and gender congruent rearing and focused on more functional outcomes. With the shift toward more patient-centered care, the Chicago Consensus strongly recommended more robust involvement of patients and families, as well as interdisciplinary experts familiar with DSD care, in guiding clinical course of treatments.

## EVOLUTION OF CLINICAL UNDERSTANDING IN DSD: CONTROVERSIES AND PROGRESS

As the scientific understanding of human development evolves, the clinical perspective tends to follow suit. Prior to and around the time of the true sex policy, the clinical approach reflected the limited understanding of gender identity, gender roles, sexuality, and sexual orientation. The policy functioned on the premise that assigning a child's gender on the basis of biological determination (e.g., external genitalia, gonads, chromosomes) would portend "normal" and heterosexual development. Along the vein of heteronormativity, there was a predilection toward ensuring heterosexual intercourse and preventing any possible desires for homosexual intercourse (Reis and Kessler 2010). For example, women with an enlarged clitoris were demonized for lack of chastity and perceived vulnerability to sexual relationships with other women. If a patient with ambiguous genitalia expressed a proclivity toward males, surgical sex assignment would gravitate toward vaginoplasty, and if the patient expressed a proclivity toward females, surgery would gravitate toward phalloplasty. As suggested by its name, the true sex policy overemphasized the biological basis (i.e., sex) of the human development process and perpetuated the importance of procreative sex in lieu of the patient's individual sexual expressions and pleasures (Kim and Kim 2012; Pasterski et al. 2010).

With the advent of the optimal gender policy, the clinical perspective turned to the nurturing aspect of care in psycho-sexual development. In order to optimize the nurturing component, the process of sex assignment for neonates with DSD began as early as possible, preferably within the first 2 years of life. The misguided, albeit well-intentioned, belief was that children with DSD would begin to cognitively label themselves as either "boy" or "girl." As a result, the clinical approach focused on facilitating that process through early and often irreversible surgical interventions in order to reduce disruption of the psychosexual development of the child.

Some of the evidence for the optimal gender policy was grounded in the aforementioned "John/Joan" case study; however, those findings were later discovered to be erroneous and the study's methodology highly unethical. There were also many flaws in the case study: by adolescence and throughout adulthood, the patient, David Reimer, disclosed that he never felt female despite his gender assignment treatments and social upbringing. In addition, the policy overlooked the growing evidence of hormonal influences in neonatal brain development vis-à-vis gender identity formation (Meyer-Bahlburg 2015; Imperato-McGinley et al. 1979; Mouriquand et al. 2016). In addition, some studies have shown that perinatal hormonal exposure may shift typically gendered behaviors, but the self-expressed gender identity of the studied population remains fixed (Imperato-McGinley et al. 1979; Rösler and Kohn 1983). In other words, although a genetically XY child with less perinatal androgen exposure may demonstrate more feminized behaviors (e.g., more reserved play, less interest in sports), through expressive testing, the child will still self-identify as a boy.

## BIOLOGICAL, PSYCHOLOGICAL, AND CULTURAL CONTEXT

Guided by the Chicago Consensus, current best practices recommend for neonates with DSD to have a comprehensive and multidisciplinary evaluation, which involves consulting with

DSD clinical experts, providing family with unbiased explanation of findings, and discussing sex assignment with the family in a culturally appropriate context (Palmer et al. 2012; Pasterski et al. 2010). For most clinical cases, sex assignment of the neonate tends to occur within the first few weeks of life. In the frame of navigating the family's cultural preferences and values, irreversible interventions, unless urgently indicated, and cosmetic surgeries relating to sex assignments are encouraged to be delayed as much as possible (Dickens 2018; Hughes et al. 2006). Some examples of urgent interventions include the construction of a urinary opening in newborns without urinary tract anomalies, removal of malignancies, or exogenous supplementation in newborns with a salt-wasting condition. The postponement of irreversible sex assignment interventions allows for a more patient-centered care, in which the child is able to offer inputs and guide subsequent courses of treatment (Meyer-Bahlburg 2011; Palmer et al. 2012). The goal of current practices is to maximize the empowerment of the patient's autonomy while still optimizing the beneficence of clinical care.

The Chicago Consensus proposed two fundamental categories of DSD—46,XX DSD and 46,XY DSD—which are subdivided into groupings based on their pathophysiology. Some common groupings of DSDs may include the following (Pasterski et al. 2010; Sandberg et al. 2017; Viau-Colindres et al. 2017):

- Chromosomal anomalies, such as Turner syndrome, Klinefelter syndrome, or sex chromosome mosaicism
- Gonadal development disorders, such as gonadal dysgenesis
- Disorders of sex anatomy, such as disorder of ovarian or testicular development
- Disorders of androgen hormone, which may lead to ambiguous genitalia development (e.g., androgen excess in congenital adrenal hyperplasia [CAH], placental aromatase deficiency), disjunction of internal or external sex anatomy (e.g., defects of androgen synthesis in 5-alpha-reductase deficiency, defects of androgen action in androgen insensitivity syndrome [AIS])

Compounding the historical binary classifications of sex, data on the true incidence of DSDs are limited. It is estimated that the overall incidence of DSDs is one in 2,000–5,500 births (Hughes et al. 2006; Kim and Kim 2012); the most common

DSDs include CAH and AIS. CAH is estimated to occur in 1 in every 10,000–15,000 live births; however, because of the high prevalence of 21-hydroxylase gene mutations in certain population, the incidence can be significantly higher: 1 in every 282 births in Yupik Eskimos in Alaska (Trakakis et al. 2009). The incidence of complete AIS is estimated to be 1 in every 20,000–64,000 XY newborns; epidemiological data on partial forms of AIS is limited (Mendoza and Motos 2013).

The public awareness about the DSD/intersex community is still slowly burgeoning. Because of the advocacy of DSD activists, there are two annual awareness days: Intersex Day of Remembrance, which falls on November 8 and generally is celebrated in Europe, and Intersex Awareness Day, which lands on October 26 and is celebrated more in anglophone countries. Some communities, such as in Australia, observe both days to bookend the two weeks of awareness for the DSD/intersex population. In addition, in 2013, the Intersex Human Rights Australia created a symbol and flag for the DSD/intersex community (Figure 7–1). The flag consists of a purple ring over a yellow background to symbolize "wholeness and completeness"; yellow was selected because it is a "hermaphrodite colour," and purple was chosen as "an intersex colour, neither blue nor pink" (Carpenter 2013).

## Questions Well-Meaning People Ask

### When treating patients, should I use "intersex" or "DSD"?

When in doubt, the best approach is to ask the individual; there is a rarely a one-size-fits-all scenario. As mentioned earlier, in the medical realm, clinicians typically use either DSD as an umbrella term or the specific medical diagnosis (e.g., congenital adrenal hyperplasia) to avoid ambiguity. In an effort to reduce stigmatization, clinicians strive to use DSD as the nomenclature for a *condition* rather than a *characteristic* of a person, that is, a person with DSD rather than a DSD person.

DSD refers to a pathophysiological condition and does not denote or necessitate a course of treatment or compulsory surgeries. On the other hand, the term intersex may reinforce the binary notion of sex and gender and can be confusing after a child receives a sex assignment—does it mean that the individual no longer has an intersex condition? For some in-

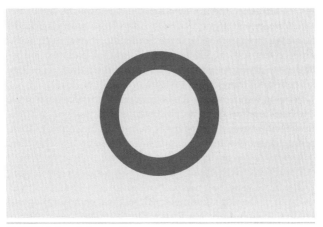

**FIGURE 7–1.** **Intersex flag.**

*Source.* Intersex Human Rights Australia, 2013. Color version available at https://ihra.org.au/22773/an-intersex-flag.

dividuals, the term intersex carries significant negative connotations along the vein of *hermaphrodite*.

At the same time, we must also balance the risk of over-medicalizing and pathologizing a vulnerable population. With the growing movement of sexual activism, some individuals preferentially self-identify as intersex for many reasons, including the following (Consortium on the Management of Disorders of Sex Development 2008):

- Some advocacy groups may express a desire to reclaim the meaning of the word intersex as a form of self-empowerment
- The term intersex can be used as an expression of gender identity akin to gender-nonbinary status
- For some individuals, the term intersex may denote a political identity, serving as a reminder of the historical discrimination the group has endured

As a result, the patient-centered approach—i.e., asking the person's preference—is recommended.

**Doesn't the word "disorder" of sex development in DSD imply there's something wrong with the person? Wouldn't that unnecessarily scare parents?**

This is an important point to deconstruct. The word *disorder* may remind this community of a long history of pathologizing. In addition, the nomenclature can complicate the disentanglement of the medical condition from an individual's identity or personhood. At the same time, the word disorder aims to improve access to medical care for patients and attempts to foster better understanding of the pathophysiology surrounding their condition (Reiner and Byne 2015).

The nomenclature is the beginning of a dialogue, not the end; seeking the advice and preference of the patient and family is the best guide in sensitively discussing the course of treatment. In fact, some DSD advocacy groups use the term *differences* or *divergence* in sex development. Along the vein of cultural sensitivity, clinicians should be aware of the Anglo/U.S.-centric aspect of medical nosology in a global context. Outside of the anglophone world, medical communities and patients may not necessarily have the same understanding of the terminology because of linguistic or cultural variations. For example, the French translation of DSD, *troubles du développement sexuel*, can be misinterpreted as disorders of sexuality development.

**Should I talk about gender dysphoria with my patient with DSD? Don't most people with DSD transition gender?**

The rates of gender transitioning may depend on the specific condition of DSD. For the most common and studied DSD condition, CAH, most patients self-identify as female and have higher rates of gender dysphoria than the general population (de Vries et al. 2007; Kreukels et al. 2018). In complete AIS, none of the participants in a study by de Vries et al. (2007) reported gender dysphoria or desired gender transitioning. In partial AIS, up to 14% of the studied participants expressed gender dysphoria and/or transitioned gender. In his Ph.D. dissertation, John Money (one of the researchers associated with the Johns Hopkins group that proposed the optimal gender policy) found that surgical interventions for sex assignment did not statistically affect the mental health of people with DSD, and overall, the studied group reported low rates of psychopathology (de Vries et al. 2007). Of note, in one of the largest cross-sectional multisite studies in the DSD population, approximately 3% of the studied population transitioned gender after puberty (in comparison with a rate of 0.2%–0.7% in the general population) (Kreukels et al. 2018). As a result, clinicians should be mindful of and curious about the exploration of potential psychological distress relating to gender identity. Furthermore, gender identity can be fluid throughout a person's life, so it is important to create an open and safe space where individuals with DSD can explore and discuss their questions and concerns.

**For people with DSD who have ambiguous genitalia, are they also transgender?**

People sometimes confuse these two groups because individuals from both groups prefer to choose their gender identity and may receive surgical interventions. Additionally, both groups challenge the social construction of binary in sex, gender identity, and gender roles and may present themselves as male, female, both, neither, or a varied combination. However, there are some important differences between the two groups. In terms of sexual morphology, people with DSD may have atypical presentation or development of external sex anatomy; on the other hand, transgender individuals, prior to their transitioning process, often have the typical appearance of their sex anatomy. Many transgender individuals experience significant gender dysphoria, which manifests from the distress of "being in a wrong body," and often self-identify as transgender. It should be noted that not everyone who is gender diverse believes they are in the "wrong body." As mentioned in an earlier section, individuals with DSD may have atypical presentation of gender roles based on their assigned sex; however, in the DSD-LIFE study of more than a thousand individuals with DSD, only about 5% reported gender changes (Kreukels et al. 2018).

**What do I say to parents when they asking, "Is it a boy or a girl?" What should families tell their friends and relatives about their child with DSD?**

The best approach is to be as culturally sensitive as possible, being honest and open with the family and their friends about the condition. It is important to acknowledge the discomfort in the uncertainty that the family is feeling and allow them time and space to process the information appropriately. In the beginning, avoiding complex medical jargon and not overloading the family with information will help them to better understand the clinical situation and process their emotions. Using nongendered language, such as "your child" or "your baby" can help destigmatize the infant's current status. The Chicago Consensus also recommends consulting an interdisciplinary team to allow families to consider different treatment options. It is important to underscore to families that gender identities can be fluid over time and that the treatment course can also evolve to reflect those changes.

# Themes That May Emerge in Therapy

## THE AMBIGUOUS SPACE OF SEX

In the intersectionality of sex, gender identity, and sexual orientation, DSD can evoke powerful feelings for individuals with DSD and their families. As some of the archaic nomenclatures (e.g., hermaphrodite, pseudo-male) may imply, individuals with DSD may feel a sense of incompleteness or lack of authenticity. It will be important to explore their understanding of what constitutes a "real boy" or a "real girl" and aspects of themselves that may feel "incomplete" or "fake." Open-ended questions such as "What feels fake or incomplete?" or "Is there a part of you that makes you feel incomplete or fake?" may help patients reflect more about their own understanding of sex development, biases, and fears.

Psychoeducation about the current scientific understanding of sex development may be helpful for some individuals. As normalized in popular culture (and typified by the obsolete true sex policy), sex is often canonized by the Y chromosome; that is to say, the presence of the Y chromosome makes a boy/man, and the absence of it creates a girl/woman. Granted, in typical development, the Y chromosome contains the testes-determining factor (TDF, formerly known as the sex-determining region), which initiates the pathway for sex characteristics associated with a male. However, the presence of the Y chromosome is not dogmatically tied to "maleness" for both biomedical and sociocultural reasons. Biomedically speaking, some researchers may suggest that sex is likely developed on a molecular, rather than chromosomal, level. With this evolving understanding of chromosomal influence, there are several exceptions to the Y chromosome and maleness rule:

1. Chromosomal changes (e.g., TDF) sometimes can be found translocated onto an X chromosome
2. Receptor sensitivity (e.g., androgen receptor) must respond appropriately to androgens in order to have masculinizing effects
3. Environmental influences (e.g., intrauterine environment, perinatal exposure to hormones) can affect the infant's physical and neuropsychological development

As implied in the discussion of their condition, individuals with DSD may have certain feelings toward their parents and families, some of which may be unacceptable to them, such as blame, anger, or hatred. It may be helpful to contextualize the patient's feelings in the interpersonal context. For example, a woman with CAH may find her virilized external genitalia unacceptable because of their morphological similarity to a penis and may be directing her frustration and anger at her genitalia toward her father.

## GENDER IDENTITY AND SEXUAL ORIENTATION

Socioculturally, on a day-to-day basis, people generally relate with one another through gender identity rather than chromosomal or molecular sex. For example, via gender identity, an individual's "maleness" is often translated into traditionally masculine behavior, appearance, and traits. It is especially important to contextualize the cultural background of the individual and potential germane political and legal ramifications. Topics associated with gender norms, such as the birth certificate or filling out the "sex" section on any legal forms, can be especially sensitive.

Some families may be tempted to ask, "Is my child going to be gay/lesbian/bisexual?" As insinuated by the optimal gender policy, some families may want to "correct the pathology" as early as possible and may express concerns about the effect of DSD on their child's future sexual orientation and gender identity. Managing expectations of the family early is instrumental because it is virtually impossible to predict an individual's future sexual orientation or gender identity.

Again, open-ended questions can be a helpful tool in facilitating a nonjudgmental forum for families to discuss their expectations. Examples include the following:

- "What would it mean to you if your son were gay?"
- "How would you feel if your daughter decides later on to change her gender?"
- "What does being a boy/man or a girl/woman mean in your family?"

For example, a family may not have fully accepted the diagnosis of DSD in the patient, and the patient's homosexuality, which is a normal variance of sexual orientation, may remind them of their child's variances in sexual morphologies.

In addition, some individuals with DSD may not necessarily self-identify as a boy or a girl. In comparison with the general population, some studies suggest that the DSD population may have a higher rate of gender nonconformity. Furthermore, a subset of those gender-nonconforming individuals may express gender dysphoric symptoms and/or seek gender-affirming medical intervention. Therapists should be mindful about exploring these topics and collaborating with the medical team as necessary and with the consent of the patient and family.

Therapists should strive to have a discussion with the family about their expectations, hopes, and fears about their child's psychosexual development as early as appropriate. For example, a family may grieve the loss of their past interpersonal relationship with the patient as a man and may fear the ambiguity of their future relationship with the patient as a woman. In addition, it may be helpful for therapists to provide further psychoeducation and to reduce the stigma surrounding the spectrum of gender identity and sexual orientation.

## FERTILITY, RELATIONSHIPS, AND FAMILY

For many individuals, having children is a natural part of life. For individuals with DSD, having children is a complicated topic mired in biological and sociocultural challenges. From a biological standpoint, therapists should be aware of the fertility barriers in the DSD population: some DSDs (e.g., Turner syndrome) carry an inherent infertility due to chromosomal abnormalities; some individuals with DSDs (e.g., Klinefelter syndrome) have significantly lower fertility in comparison with the general population; and other individuals with DSDs (e.g., partial AIS) may have lost fertility because of necessary gonadectomies to mitigate malignancy risks.

For individuals with fertility challenges, loss (e.g., loss of normalcy, loss of ability to be a biological parent) may be a prominent theme, which can serve as a powerful and painful reminder of their condition. Adults who received irreversible interventions during infancy or childhood may feel particularly helpless because they were unable to participate in those clinical decisions, or they may even feel anger at their parents for consenting to those treatments. In addition, therapists should be mindful that the patient's partners may not be fully aware of the patient's diagnosis. Individuals who have the possibility of fertility (e.g., people with CAH) may have to grapple with the possibility of passing on their condition to their children. Because DSDs encompass a wide range of genetic anomalies, the pattern of inheritance can be autosomal dominant, autosomal recessive, X-linked, or varied manner based on the involved gene(s).

If the patient does bring up the topic of fertility, children, or parenthood, the therapist may explore further the significance and meaning behind their desires by asking the following questions:

- "What does being a parent signify to you?"
- "What does the word *family* mean to you?"
- "Having a biological child can be important to many people. How does it feel for you?"

The therapist can work with an endocrinologist or reproductive specialist to assist individuals with DSD who may wish to examine reproductive technologies, such as, sperm aspiration, in vitro fertilization, and surrogacy.

## NORMALCY, TRUTH, AND SHAME

At birth, one of the most common questions from families to their providers is "Is it a boy or a girl?" It is also one of the most common questions for families to receive from their friends and loved ones. After hearing the DSD diagnosis, families understandably are often shocked that something atypical and unexpected has occurred to their child and may be worried about their child's future. In addition, gender norms are socially ingrained in the celebrations of pregnancy (e.g., the naming process, gender reveal parties) and birth (e.g., pink or blue themed clothing, gendered toys). For many families, the ambiguity surrounding their child's sex and gender identity can evoke an immense feeling of shame in the gendered social celebrations and a loss of the feeling of or hope for normalcy they have imagined in the prenatal and perinatal periods. Finally, because many languages are gendered, the family may feel a literal and metaphorical speechlessness in talking about their child.

During this period, therapists can work with the medical team to provide a forum for the family to ask questions, express their confusion and concerns, and reflect on their intense emotions. This crucial process allows the family to avoid the pitfall of developing shame- and secrecy-based be-haviors toward their child. An explicit and transparent nor-malizing statement that acknowledges the family's shame can free them to express their complex emotions. Examples of such statement include the following:

- "It can be really stressful and scary to hear that something unexpected has happened to your child."
- "Some families may feel embarrassed and uncomfortable that their child wasn't the little girl they had dreamed of."
- "It can feel shameful to not know what to say when others ask about the gender of your child."

It is equally important to recognize and clarify the parents' subconscious wish that their negative emotions will be fixed by the child's cosmetic surgeries. In addition, by creating a cul-ture of openness from the beginning, the family will be better able to support their child and help the child avoid internaliza-tion of shame and feelings of alienation. The manner in which families disclose to others may also shape how the child ap-proaches disclosures to friends and partners in the future. Many families will also benefit from peer support groups to es-tablish a sense of community and mutual advocacy.

Another scenario in which the family and the patient seek psychotherapeutic care may include adolescents with DSD who were not aware of their diagnosis growing up. For some cases of DSD without ambiguous sex anatomy or overt med-ical complications, the official diagnosis may occur around the time of puberty, when sex hormones become pertinent. For example, an adolescent patient with complete AIS may present to their pediatrician for amenorrhea.

When possible, the medical team should work with a ther-apist specializing in DSD care to disclose the diagnosis in order to facilitate the aforementioned process of understanding DSD's biopsychosocial impacts. A therapeutic disclosure should be 1) complete and transparent; 2) geared toward the entire family, which may include the patient, the parents, and loved ones; and 3) tailored appropriately for the developmental age of the child. It is important to acknowledge and process po-tential immature defenses within the family, such as denial, in-tellectualization, and reaction formation. Some families may object to disclosing the DSD diagnosis to the child. The thera-pist may validate the concern surrounding the sensitivity of the topic and concurrently explain to the family about empowering the patient. Some examples include the following statement:

- "This diagnosis may be surprising and may bring up strong emotions in everyone."
- "I understand that you want to protect your child from feeling hurt; however, children often look to their parents on how to navigate a challenge."
- "We want to show your child that you still love him no matter what and to empower your child by showing him that his condition doesn't completely define him."

The goal of care is similar to neonatal cases: processing and deconstructing the stigma and shame surrounding the DSD condition.

## Conclusion

In the intersectionality of sex, gender identity, and sexual orientation, intersex considerations may evoke powerful emotions for patients and their families. By providing a nonjudgmental therapeutic space and asking open-ended questions, clinicians can encourage patients to safely explore potential conscious and unconscious psychological distress. Current best practices recommend for neonates with disorder of sex development (DSD) to have a comprehensive and multidisciplinary evaluation, which involves consulting with DSD clinical experts, providing family with unbiased explanation of findings, and discussing sex assignment with the family in a culturally appropriate context. Given this vulnerable community's history of medical pathologization, clinicians should strive to destigmatize care by tailoring nomenclature in medical documentation on the basis of individual and family preferences.

## FIVE TAKE-HOME POINTS

- Individuals with disorder of sex development (DSD) face challenges at the intersection of sex, gender identity, and sexual orientation.
- In working with the DSD population, sensitivity surrounding nomenclature and gendered language is paramount

in order to reduce stigma for a vulnerable minority population that historically has been pathologized by the medical community.

- Current best practices recommend that neonates with
  DSD have a comprehensive and multidisciplinary evaluation, which involves consulting with DSD clinical experts, providing the family with unbiased explanation of
  findings, and discussing sex assignment with the family
  in a culturally appropriate context.

- In the frame of navigating the family's cultural preferences and values, it is recommended that irreversible
  medical interventions, unless urgently indicated, and
  cosmetic surgeries relating to sex assignment be delayed
  as much as possible.

- Given the wide range of DSDs, a patient-centered approach in clinical care is highly recommended: When in
  doubt, ask and work with the patient and family.

## Resources

Accord Alliance, www.accordalliance.org. This website hosts
  clinical guidelines for DSD for providers and families.
interACT, http://interactadvocates.org. InterACT is a youth-
  led advocacy program for intersex teens and twentysome-
  things to come together, share experiences, and raise intersex
  awareness.
International Lesbian, Gay, Bisexual, Trans, and Intersex Association, https://ilga.org. The website has numerous
  branches across the world and lists some local resources
  for LGBTQI individuals not living in the North American
  continent.
Intersex Initiative, www.ipdx.org. This group is based primarily in the Pacific Northwest and Japan. The website
  has a variety of publications and articles about DSD culture and patient experiences.
Intersex Society of North America, www.isna.org. Founded
  in 1993, this group is one of the largest support groups for
  individuals with DSD.
Intersex support and advocacy groups, https://interact
  advocates.org/resources/intersex-organizations. This
  website from interACT contains a comprehensive list of

support groups and organizations specifically based on DSD conditions.

# References

Carpenter M: An intersex flag. Newtown, NSW, Australia, Intersex Human Rights Australia, 2013. Available at: https://ihra.org.au/22773/an-intersex-flag. Accessed March 31, 2019.

Consortium on the Management of Disorders of Sex Development: Clinical Guidelines for the Management of Disorders of Sex Development in Childhood. Whitehouse Station, NJ, Accord Alliance, 2008

de Vries ALC, Doreleijers TAH, Cohen-Kettenis PT: Disorders of sex development and gender identity outcome in adolescence and adulthood: understanding gender identity development and its clinical implications. Pediatr Endocrinol Rev 4(4):343–351, 2007 17643082

Dickens BM: Management of intersex newborns: legal and ethical developments. Int J Gynaecol Obstet 143(2):255–259, 2018 29943821

Hughes IA, Houk C, Ahmed SF, et al: Consensus statement on management of intersex disorders. Arch Dis Child 91(7):554–563, 2006 16624884

Imperato-McGinley J, Peterson RE, Gautier T, et al: Androgens and the evolution of male-gender identity among male pseudohermaphrodites with 5alpha-reductase deficiency. N Engl J Med 300(22):1233–1237, 1979 431680

Kim KS, Kim J: Disorders of sex development. Korean J Urol 53(1):1–8, 2012 22323966

Kreukels BPC, Köhler B, Nordenström A, et al: Gender dysphoria and gender change in disorders of sex development/intersex conditions: results From the DSD-LIFE study. J Sex Med 15(5):777–785, 2018 29606626

Mendoza N, Motos MA: Androgen insensitivity syndrome. Gynecol Endocrinol 29(1):1–5, 2013 22812659

Meyer-Bahlburg HFL: Gender assignment and reassignment in 46,XY pseudohermaphroditism and related conditions. J Clin Endocrinol Metab 84(10):3455–3458, 1999 10522979

Meyer-Bahlburg HFL: Gender monitoring and gender reassignment of children and adolescents with a somatic disorder of sex development. Child Adolesc Psychiatr Clin N Am 20(4):639–649, 2011 22051002

Meyer-Bahlburg HFL: Commentary on Kraus' (2015) "classifying intersex in DSM-5: critical reflections on gender dysphoria." Arch Sex Behav 44(7):1737–1740, 2015 26168979

Money J, Hampson JG, Hampson JL: Hermaphroditism: recommendations concerning assignment of sex, change of sex and psychologic management. Bull Johns Hopkins Hosp 97(4):284–300, 1955 13260819

Mouriquand PD, Gorduza DB, Gay CL, et al: Surgery in disorders of sex development (DSD) with a gender issue: if (why), when, and how? J Pediatr Urol 12(3):139–149, 2016 27132944

Palmer BW, Wisniewski AB, Schaeffer TL, et al: A model of delivering multi-disciplinary care to people with 46 XY DSD. J Pediatr Urol 8(1):7–16, 2012 22078657

Pasterski V, Prentice P, Hughes IA: Consequences of the Chicago consensus on disorders of sex development (DSD): current practices in Europe. Arch Dis Child 95(8):618–623, 2010 19773218

Reiner W, Byne W: Interview with William Reiner, MD, urologist and child psychiatrist, on approaches to care for individuals with disorders of sex development and somatic intersex conditions. LGBT Health 2(1):3–10, 2015 26790011

Reis E, Kessler S: Why history matters: fetal dex and intersex. Am J Bioeth 10(9):58–59, 2010 20818565

Rösler A, Kohn G: Male pseudohermaphroditism due to 17 beta-hydroxysteroid dehydrogenase deficiency: studies on the natural history of the defect and effect of androgens on gender role. J Steroid Biochem 19(1B):663–674, 1983 6310248

Sandberg DE, Gardner M, Callens N, et al: Interdisciplinary care in disorders/differences of sex development (DSD): the psychosocial component of the DSD-translational research network. Am J Med Genet C Semin Med Genet 175(2):279–292, 2017 28574671

Trakakis E, Basios G, Trompoukis P, et al: An update to 21-hydroxylase deficient congenital adrenal hyperplasia. Gynecol Endocrinol 26(1):63–71, 2009 19499408

Viau-Colindres J, Axelrad M, Karaviti LP, et al: Bringing back the term "intersex." Pediatrics 140(5):e20170505, 2017 29070532

# Chapter 8

# Asexual

## The First A in LGBTQ²IAPA

SELALE GUNAL
PETROS LEVOUNIS, M.D., M.A.

> I'm not gay. I mean, I don't think I am, but…I don't think
> I'm straight, either. I don't know what I am.
> I think I might be nothing.
>
> —*Todd Chavez*, BoJack Horseman

## Psychological and Cultural Context

The term *asexual* has been known as the mode of reproduction in single-cell organisms since the nineteenth-century work of Gregor Mendel, but for the past 15 years the term has also been used for human sexuality. Many people are unaware that asexuality exists or believe that it is not real. A basic definition of asexuality is the lack of sexual attraction. Asexuality can be contrasted with the term *allosexual*, which refers to someone who experiences sexual attraction. Use of these two terms helps counteract the implication that asexuality is abnormal. Correct understanding of sexual diversity will help clinicians offer support for people frequently criticized and hurt by misunderstanding of their sexuality.

### HISTORY

The lack of sexual attraction was first described in 1948 by Alfred Kinsey as *category X* in a study that classified the sexual behavior of interviewed subjects (Kinsey et al. 1948) (Figure

| | Kinsey model |
|---|---|
| 0 | Exclusively heterosexual |
| 1 | Predominantly heterosexual |
| 2 | Predominantly heterosexual (more than incidentallly) |
| 3 | Equally heterosexual and homosexual |
| 4 | Predominantly homosexual (more than incidentally) |
| 5 | Predominantly homosexual |
| 6 | Exclusively homosexual |
| Category X | No sociosexual reactions |

FIGURE 8–1. **Kinsey sexuality orientation scale.**

*Source.* Adapted from Kinsey et al. 1948.

8–1). Several decades later, Michael Storms proposed a model whose matrix included asexuality as one of four categories of sexual attraction (Storms 1980) (Figure 8–2). However, statistical prevalence studies have emerged only during the last 10–15 years. Bogaert's (2004) analysis of data from 18,000 British individuals, based on self-identification ("I have never felt sexually attracted to anyone"), and other population studies in the United States (Lippa 2017) indicate that approximately 1% of the population self identifies as asexual.

With the creation of the Asexual Visibility and Education Network (AVEN) in 2001, awareness of the asexual community has increased. The Acebook, an asexual dating and social networking site, was created in 2008 by an AVEN member, offering another forum for asexual people to connect with each other. Many individuals first learn about and explore their asexuality through online communities such as Tumblr, personal sites, and blogs. Recently, several television shows, including *BoJack Horseman* and *Shadowhunters*, and news articles have explored the topic of asexuality (Ghaleb 2018). A 2011 documentary film, *(A)sexual*, successfully informed audiences what asexuality looks like. However, asexuality is still a very little known or accepted identity.

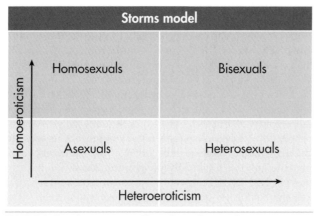

FIGURE 8–2. **Storms sexuality orientation scale.**
*Source.* Adapted from Storms 1980.

## CATEGORIZATION

Asexuality has been defined differently by various researchers, with characteristics that include the following:

1. Lack of sexual behavior
2. Sexual dysfunction or low sexual excitation
3. Psychiatric condition
4. All or some of the above

However, it is important to note what asexuality is not: Asexuality cannot be considered a psychiatric condition. Prior to DSM-5 (American Psychiatric Association 2013), asexuality would have been considered a hypoactive sexual desire disorder (HSDD). Asexuality is different from HSDD and sexual aversion disorder, which was removed from DSM-5 because of its rarity and a lack of evidence. HSDD is a medical illness, whereas asexuality establishes a social identity. Research on the nature of asexuality supports asexuality as an orientation and suggests that rates of psychiatric symptoms may not differ significantly between self-identified asexuals and the general population. For example, Brotto et al. (2015) found no difference in anxiety or negative affect between asexual and nonasexual women when viewing erotic films.

DSM-5 includes wording that clearly recognizes asexuality: "If a lifelong lack of sexual desire is better explained by

*Asexual*                                                                                   **147**

one's self-identification as 'asexual,' then a diagnosis of female sexual interest/arousal disorder would not be made"
(American Psychiatric Association 2013, p. 434). "If the man's
low desire is explained by self-identification as an asexual,
then a diagnosis of male hypoactive sexual desire disorder is
not made" (American Psychiatric Association 2013, p. 443).

Many people often confuse celibacy with asexuality. *Celibacy*
is the conscious decision not to have sex. Asexual people may be
celibate as well, but they can also be sexually active. Asexual
people may choose to have sex for any number of reasons, including wanting to please or be intimate with a partner or simply to enjoy the physically pleasurable sensation sex can
provide. Essentially, being celibate does not make a person asexual, and having sex does not make someone allosexual. Many
asexual people also identify as being sex repulsed, meaning
they personally are averse to the idea of having sex. Other asexual people may consider themselves indifferent and, as mentioned previously, could be open to the idea of having sex.

Some asexual people also identify as *aromantic*, or not experiencing romantic attraction. Others identify only as asexual
and have an *alloromantic* (i.e., not aromantic) identity, such as
*homoromantic*, a person who is romantically attracted to a
member of the same sex, or *biromantic*, a person who is attracted to both males and females romantically (Figure 8–3).
This method of self-identification uses the *split attraction model*,
which essentially states that romantic and sexual attraction are
distinct from each other. For example, someone might say they
are aromantic asexual (or "aroace" for shorter), or they may
say they are gay asexual if they experience romantic attraction.

The split attraction model is used primarily by the asexual and aromantic community. For most other people in the
LGBTQ+ community, their sexual and romantic identities co-
incide with each other, but aromantic and asexual people
seem to experience more variation, so asexual people often
specify their romantic orientation as well. There is currently
little to no scientific research on the split attraction model, on
whether it is a valid way of expressing variations in sexual
identity, or why it seems that split attraction occurs mainly
within the asexual community.

## RESEARCH

Existing scientific research on asexuality, including the older
studies by Kinsey et al. (1948) and Storms (1980) (see Figures

| Romantic orientation | Sexual orientation: Asexual | Sexual orientation: Heterosexual | Sexual orientation: Homosexual | Sexual orientation: Bi/pansexual |
|---|---|---|---|---|
| Aromantic | no sexual or romantic attraction | sexual attraction to another sex but little or no romantic attraction | sexual attraction to same sex but no romantic attraction | sexual attraction to all sexes but no romantic attraction |
| Heteroromantic | no sexual attraction or romantic attraction to another sex | | | |
| Homoromantic | no sexual attraction or romantic attraction to same sex | | | |
| Bi/panromantic | no sexual attraction or romantic attraction to all sexes | | | |

FIGURE 8–3. **Patterns of romantic orientation based on sexual attraction.**

**TABLE 8–1.** Asexuality identification scale items

Sexual attraction/desire

Masturbation

Sexual fantasy

Erotica

Sexual activity

Sexual identity

Sex-related disgust

Self-reported sexual arousal

Inability to relate to others' sexuality

Sexual interest

Sexual avoidance

Relationships

Romantic attraction and intimacy

*Source.* Yule et al. 2015.

8–1 and 8–2), suggests that asexual individuals in general are capable of sexual stimulation and arousal but do not initiate or pursue sex (McConaghy 1994). This research made asexuality culturally visible. More recent studies, which were based mainly on surveys (Prause and Graham 2007; Scherrer 2008), improved the understanding of the prevalence of asexuality and concluded that each individual has their personal narratives and interpretations of their asexual identity. These survey-based studies also attempted to classify participants into better-defined groups. Specifically, Yule et al. (2015) and Brotto et al. (2015) developed a reliable, neutral self-report measure of asexuality consisting of 13 concepts (Table 8–1).

The argument can be made that categorization of asexuality is unnecessary and may limit the advancement of identity and community-focused explorations. However, categorization allows researchers to recruit more representative individuals of the asexual population, which would support an increased understanding of asexuality. In addition to the concepts in Table 8–1, community efforts also add to the description and classification of asexuality. Terms such as gray asexual, gray sexual, and demisexual can be used to describe individuals identified with the area between asexuality and sexuality. For example, a gray-sexual person may experience sexual attraction very rarely, only under specific circumstances, or of an intensity so low that it can be ignored. A gray-sexual person may date a lot of people but view only one or two of them as sexy.

Researchers in this field also attempt to understand the distinction between sexual attraction and romantic attraction. The neurological basis for sexual and romantic attraction is not exactly the same, but both have many common components. Specifically, several of the neurochemicals that mediate mammalian bonding and romantic love—oxytocin, vasopressin, and dopamine—also mediate sexual behavior. Both romantic love and sexual desire require complex involvement of diverse brain areas that include mainly the reward system. However, romantic love and sexual desire do not have the same goal orientation, which has been shown by differences in brain activation patterns (Aron et al. 2005). In human functional magnetic resonance imaging studies, the brain regions that showed distinctive patterns of activity when viewing romantic partners did not overlap with regions typically activated during sexual arousal (Aron et al. 2005; Diamond and Amso 2008).

## CURRENT ISSUES

As mentioned in the subsection "History," most people first find out about asexuality online. Most asexual terms and identities, including the community flag and subcategories of the identity, have been developed online. The Asexual Community Survey reports that Tumblr was the first community in which a significant number (39%) of asexual respondents participated (Ace Community Survey Team 2016; Bauer et al. 2018). Today, some anecdotal reports claim that Tumblr can be a hostile environment for asexual people, depending on which communities they view or engage with.

Most LGBTQ communities and organizations other than some online communities (e.g., Reddit, Tumblr) consider asexual people to be part of the LGBTQ+ community. Almost every LGBTQ+ organization, such as the Trevor Project, accepts asexuality as a part of the LGBTQ community. However, in recent years, there have been debates online, especially on Tumblr, about whether asexual people should actually be included. Exclusionists—people who do not think asexual people are a part of the LGBTQ community—say that same-sex attraction is what defines whether or not any identity is LGBTQ. They feel that asexuality is not inherently LGBT because asexual people do not experience attraction and think asexual people should be included only if they are also gay, bisexual, or panromantic. Some people think that asexual people, especially if they are heteroromantic, gray, or demisexual, are "basically straight" and therefore should not be included. Hostility and rejection as a person's first experience with the asexual community, and the LGBTQ community as a whole, can be harmful to young people who are just discovering asexuality and exploring their own identity.

## Questions Well-Meaning People Ask

**Am I asexual?**

Asexuality simply refers to individuals who do not feel sexual attraction. However, asexuality is a general term that lots of different people in different circumstances use. What is essential is what feels right for an individual. If you feel that you don't experience sexual attraction, you may be asexual. The only person who can determine if you are asexual is you. It is also important to remember that sexuality is fluid, and you can change how you identify at any point in your life.

**How can I know if I'm asexual without having sex?**

Allosexual people figure out their orientation through crushes they have when they are young. Asexuality is harder to figure out because you are looking for something that isn't there. However, similar to allosexuals, many asexual people are able to figure out their orientation without having sex first. Many asexual people recall feelings of confusion when other people discussed crushes, even thinking that maybe everyone else was simply making it up. Many people find it difficult to determine if they are asexual simply because they don't know that the term even exists. After realizing that asexuality actually exists and learning about it, some asexual people say they feel that the identity just "fits."

**Is there something wrong with me?**

No. Although many asexual people do feel "broken" or as if something is lacking, especially because of how much emphasis is placed on sex is in our society, asexual people are not broken. You do not need to experience sexual attraction in order to have healthy and fulfilling relationships.

**Isn't asexuality just a phase? Aren't asexual people just late bloomers?**

No. Asexuality is a real sexuality. That being said, it is possible that people may change their identity over the course of their lifetime. Someone who used to identify as asexual may change their identity to gray or demisexual, or even to an allosexual identity, later on. This does not mean, however, that their asexuality was a phase. Calling asexuality a phase implies that everyone who identifies as asexual will change their identity as they get older, which is not the case.

**Is asexuality a psychiatric disorder?**

No. However, distress associated with any sexuality, including asexuality, may cause psychiatric symptoms. Although therapists should never "diagnose" someone as asexual, they evaluate and treat asexual people for psychological distress and full psychiatric conditions just as they would for people who are heterosexual, gay, bisexual, transgender, or queer. In addition, they provide the tools and information for their patients to make sense of their sexuality and improve their interpersonal relationships, as crystal clear or messy as these may be.

**Is asexuality caused by trauma?**

There is no evidence that asexuality is caused by trauma, abuse, or sexual assault. There are certainly asexual people who have experienced trauma, just as there are in any community, but it cannot be said that their trauma caused, or is even associated with, their asexuality.

**Is asexuality a sexual dysfunction?**

A study by Brotto and Yule (2011) showed no difference in genital arousal patterns between asexual and sexual women when presented with sexual triggers. Asexuality is different from sexual desire disorder, which requires the experience of clinically significant personal distress. A recent study of 400 men and women comparing individuals with sexual desire disorder and asexuality also confirmed that asexuality differs from sexual dysfunction (Brotto and Yule 2017). The study showed that compared with asexual individuals, individuals who met diagnostic criteria for HSDD were significantly more likely to engage in sexual intercourse or sexual fantasy and had higher levels of sexual desire and sex-related distress.

**Can asexual people date and be in romantic relationships?**

Yes. Asexual people may be in romantic relationships with asexual or allosexual people. As long as there is open communication and understanding of boundaries, there is no reason why an asexual person could not be in a romantic relationship. The asexual community has also developed the term *queer/quasi platonic relationship* (QPR) to describe a relationship that is between friendship and dating. Many asexual people prefer QPRs over traditional dating. QPRs are not "just friendships"; they involve a bond that is somewhere between platonic feelings and romantic/sexual attraction and may or may not include sex or romantic actions such as hugging and kissing. What a QPR is, or even if a relationship is a QPR, is determined by the people in the relationship and what they are comfortable with.

**My child came out to me as asexual. How can I support them?**

Acknowledge and validate their identity. Do not tell them that 1) it may just be a phase, 2) they are too young to know, or 3) they just haven't found the right person yet. Although any of these statements may end up being true, trivializing your child's asexuality (or any sexuality for that matter) can be harmful and informs the child that you don't truly accept their identity. Coming out takes a lot of courage, especially when asexuality is not common, not commonly known, not commonly accepted, and often not even considered a real sexuality.

Another way you can support your child is to research asexuality on your own. Most asexual people coming out do not expect people to know what they mean when they say they are asexual and are prepared to explain. Although there is enough published information now that asexual people shouldn't be required to give a presentation every time they come out, most of them are happy to do so.

# Themes that May Emerge in Therapy

Asexual people often feel as if they are broken or abnormal. They may have been told that sex is a natural part of life or a basic aspect of being human, leading them to feel like a freak or even inhuman. They may hate being asexual, wanting instead to be "normal."

## ADOLESCENCE

In many parts of the world, teenagers are expected to start having romantic and sexual experiences. Asexual teenagers may feel left out from the experiences of their peers, or they may feel pressured to be in a relationship or encouraged to have sex when they do not want to.

## COMING OUT

The process of coming out for most people who belong to minority sexual orientations is not easy as the individuals try to find acceptance both from partners and from themselves. Because science and information on asexuality are not well established, asexual individuals may require more awareness and support from their peers for their sexuality than do individuals with other sexual orientations.

Feeling a lack of sexual attraction to others is deemed to be outside of the norm and is not well understood by those who do experience sexual attractions. Although some people refuse to believe in its existence, asexuality is a recognized and legitimate sexual orientation, and coming out as such is an important part of self-acceptance and understanding and celebrating one's humanity.

## DATING

Asexual people may fear that they are unlovable and that they won't be able to have intimate relationships. Many asexual people date. Sexual activity is not necessary for a relationship. Asexuals may have meaningful relationships and enjoy intimacy and closeness.

## MENTAL HEALTH AND ILLNESS

Asexuality is characterized as a lack of sexual attraction, which is different from a sexual dysfunction. However, some drugs may produce the side effect of a lack of sexual desire, which can lead to diagnosis of substance/medication-induced sexual dysfunction (American Psychiatric Association 2013, pp. 446–450). Medication-induced lack of sexual desire is not a sexuality because it is not an innate and stable characteristic, but it may be mistaken for asexuality (Gupta 2017). This aspect of asexuality must be considered in therapies.

Although there is no evidence that the rates of psychiatric disorders are significantly different between self-identified asexual individuals and the general population (Brotto et al. 2015), a recent survey-based research study suggested a higher rate of asexuality among individuals with autism spectrum disorder (ASD; George and Stokes 2018). In this study, rates of ASD were higher among homosexual, bisexual, and asexual individuals than heterosexual individuals. The results highlight a need for specialized sex education programs and additional support for ASD populations.

## SEX

Asexual people are frequently stereotyped as being cold and unfeeling, but being uninterested in sex doesn't automatically make an individual distant or emotionally unavailable. Some asexual people may want to have some form of sex, but they typically have difficulty talking about that sexual activity with a partner, and at times they may feel pressured to perform more traditional sexual activities.

## Conclusion

Although our understanding of asexuality is still incomplete, we now appreciate asexuality as a legitimate sexual orientation separate from a disorder. Additional scientific research, clinical competence, and cultural awareness of asexuality are greatly needed in order to effectively and compassionately care for people who identify with this sexual orientation minority.

## FIVE TAKE-HOME POINTS

- Asexuality is a sexual orientation; it includes many variations, including gray sexuality and demisexuality.
- Although some asexual people may enjoy sex, not being interested in pursuing sex is normal in asexuality.

- Asexuality is not a disorder, but the boundary between a sexual desire disorder and asexuality is not currently well defined.

- Asexuality is distinct from aromanticity. People may be both asexual and aromantic or only one of the two.

- Individuals who identify as asexual may experience distress and may need psychological or psychiatric support, not unlike other sexual minority or heterosexual populations.

# Resources

The Asexual Visibility and Education Network (AVEN), www.asexuality.org

The Trevor Project Support Center: Asexual, www.thetrevor project.org/trvr_support_center/asexual/#sm.00000301 wiwvjbfdoxvrn22xfnilg

Ace Week (asexual awareness), www.asexualawareness week.com/index.html

# References

Ace Community Survey Team: The Ace Community Survey, 2016. Available at: https://asexualcensus.wordpress.com. Accessed February 5, 2020.

American Psychiatric Association: Diagnostic and Statistical Manual of Mental Disorders, 5th Edition. Arlington, VA, American Psychiatric Association, 2013

Aron A, Fisher H, Mashek DJ, et al: Reward, motivation, and emotion systems associated with early stage intense romantic love. J Neurophysiol 94(1):327–337, 2005 15928068

Bauer C, Miller T, Ginoza M, et al: Initial participation, in 2016 Asexual Community Survey. Asexual Visibility and Education Network, November 15, 2018. Available at: https://asexualcensus.files.word press.com/2018/11/2016_ace_community_survey_report.pdf. Accessed February 5, 2020.

Bogaert AF: Asexuality: prevalence and associated factors in a national probability sample. J Sex Res 41(3):279–287, 2004 15497056

Brotto LA, Yule MA: Physiological and subjective sexual arousal in self-identified asexual women. Arch Sex Behav 40(4):699–712, 2011 20857185

Brotto LA, Yule MA: Asexuality: sexual orientation, paraphilia, sexual dysfunction, or none of the above? Arch Sex Behav 46(3):619–627, 2017 27542079

Brotto LA, Yule MA, Gorzalka BB: Asexuality: an extreme variant of sexual desire disorder? J Sex Med 12(3):646–660, 2015 25545124

Diamond A, Amso D: Contributions of neuroscience to our understanding of cognitive development. Curr Dir Psychol Sci 17(2):136–141, 2008 18458793

George R, Stokes MA: Sexual orientation in autism spectrum disorder. Autism Res 11(1):133–141, 2018 29159906

Ghaleb S: Asexuality is still hugely misunderstood. TV is slowly changing that. Vox, March 26, 2018. Available at: www.vox.com/culture/2018/3/26/16291562/asexuality-tv-history-bojack-shadowhunters-game-of-thrones. Accessed May 15, 2019.

Gupta K: What does asexuality teach us about sexual disinterest? Recommendations for health professionals based on a qualitative study with asexually identified people. J Sex Marital Ther 43(1):1–14, 2017 26643598

Kinsey AC, Pomeroy WR, Martin CE: Sexual Behavior in the Human Male. Philadelphia, PA, WB Saunders, 1948

Lippa RA: Category specificity of self-reported sexual attraction and viewing times to male and female models in a large U.S. sample: sex, sexual orientation, and demographic effects. Arch Sex Behav 46(1):167–178, 2017 27730412

McConaghy N: Biologic theories of sexual orientation. Arch Gen Psychiatry 51(5):431–432, 1994

Prause N, Graham CA: Asexuality: classification and characterization. Arch Sex Behav 36(3):341–356, 2007 17345167

Scherrer KS: Coming to an asexual identity: negotiating identity, negotiating desire. Sexualities 11(5):621–641, 2008 20593009

Storms MD: Theories of sexual orientation. J Pers Soc Psychol 38(5):783–792, 1980

Yule MA, Brotto LA, Gorzalka BB: A validated measure of no sexual attraction: the Asexuality Identification Scale. Psychol Assess 27(1):148–160, 2015 25383584

# Chapter 9

# Pansexual

## *The P in LGBTQ²IAPA*

VICTORIA FORMOSA, L.C.S.W.

> I just like people.
> I'm more attracted to personalities rather than genders.
> But I'm still not 100% sure about labeling myself.
>
> —*Participant in study by Galupo et al. 2016*

## Psychological and Cultural Context

The most common definition of *pansexuality* is "individuals who feel they are sexually, emotionally, and spiritually capable of being attracted to any person regardless of gender or sex" (Belous and Bauman 2017, p. 58). *Sex* refers to the genitals that someone has. *Gender* is the way that someone identifies and expresses themself in terms of masculinity and femininity. The prefix *pan* means "all" in Latin. A person who identifies as pansexual can be attracted to all different types of people, and their attraction is not restricted to people of one gender or sex. An important piece of the pansexual identity is the idea that genitals do not have to be the most important part of attraction. For many pansexual people, genitals and gender are not top priorities when they are seeking relationships. Pansexual people are open to relationships with anyone they feel connected to. The word *all* means that pansexual people are open to all possibilities for love and attraction between consenting adults. The word *all* is especially important because it emphasizes that there are more than two genders and more than two sexes. Gender and sex are multidimensional and are unique to every person.

Learning about pansexuality can be confusing for people who have not been exposed to gender diversity before. Sexuality in and of itself can be a complicated thing to explain. It is made even more difficult when the people who first teach us about sexuality are usually parents or health teachers who are not completely comfortable with the topic themselves. In order to make such conversations easier, these adults often use a tool they think will simplify things: the binary. The binary defines one thing in opposition to another and helps people organize the world. Some examples of the binary include right or wrong, good or bad, healthy or unhealthy, penis or vagina, man or woman, and gay or straight. When someone explains gender and sex using the binary, they typically explain that a person is born with either a penis or a vagina and thus is either a man or a woman. The binary gives us only two options to choose from instead of having to consider a variety of options. When things are explained in a binary way, there is no room for a gray area.

In the first part of this chapter, we briefly focus on how sex, gender, and sexuality are defined through binary terms. This is typically how we learn about sexuality. Next, we describe ways in which sex, gender and sexuality can be understood in nonbinary terms. We then attempt to define how pansexual people see sexuality. Pansexual people are a diverse group, and each pansexual person will have a unique way of defining their own sexuality. Finally, we explore some realities for pansexual people and some common challenges that they face. Learning more about the vastness of gender, sex, and sexuality is not only crucial to understanding pansexual people but also will help clinicians better understand themselves.

## Sex, Gender, and Sexuality in Binary Terms

When people look at sex, gender, and sexuality through a binary lens, definitions are drastically oversimplified. Because there are only two options, binary thinking fails to truly recognize and define the multidimensional nature of human sex, gender, and sexuality. An explanation of sex, gender, and sexual orientation in binary terms looks something like this: People are born with penises or vaginas, they are men or women, they are masculine or feminine, and they are gay or straight. If someone is born with a penis, he is a man, and he will be expected to express his gender in a way that is deemed masculine by his culture.

Bisexuality can exist in binary terms because it can be defined as someone who is attracted to both men and women. When looking at bisexuality through a binary lens, it is still with the understanding that there are *only* men and women, penises and vaginas, masculine and feminine. As explained later in the section "Questions Well-Meaning People Ask," the definition of bisexuality changes when one uses a nonbinary lens.

## Sex, Gender, and Sexual Orientation in Nonbinary Terms

Thinking in a nonbinary way opens up a world of possibility. When people view the world in nonbinary terms, they no longer expect people to fit into one of two boxes. All bodies and identities are valid regardless of whether or not they conform to binary standards. Instead of two options, there are as many options for sex, gender, and sexuality as there are people in the world.

Genitals should not dictate a person's gender or the pronouns we use to refer to people. Genitals are not binary because there are more possibilities than simply penises and vaginas. People are born with a variety of different genitals that do not conform to the penis/vagina binary. In addition, people who are born with penises do not necessarily grow up to identify as men. Someone born with a penis might identify as a woman. Someone born with a penis might not feel particularly drawn to either label of man or woman and can identify as nonbinary. Nonbinary people do not conform to strictly masculine or feminine gender expressions. They may express themselves in an androgynous way; they may play with different gender expressions based on how they feel on any given day.

When thinking in nonbinary terms, there can be no such thing as "opposite sex" because opposite implies there are only two options. People can still be heterosexual, homosexual, and bisexual but these are not the only options. This is where pansexuality comes in. Pansexual people acknowledge that there are an endless number of gender identities and more than two options for genitals. They are open to the possibility of being attracted to any consenting adult regardless of their genitals or gender identity. Pansexual people reject the emphasis put on genitals and gender identity in attraction. Genitals and gender identity are not priorities in choosing a romantic or intimate partner. Because they reject the binary, pansexual people do not define their sexuality in opposition to other sexualities. This is why binary language will not help you understand pansexual people.

Binary thinking is simple, easy to understand, and easy to explain. This is because there are only a handful of options for sex, gender, and sexual orientation. It is also because most of us were taught about sexuality in a binary way. If we grew up being taught about the complexity of sexuality, bodies, and gender identities, pansexuality might be easier to understand.

Practice letting go of the rigidity that comes along with the traditional understanding of sexuality. Intersex, transgender, nonbinary, and pansexual people exist. We cannot ignore them. Ask yourself, "What would it be like for me to let go of the binary?" It may be confusing and overwhelming at first, but in time it may be a relief to accept that you are not restricted to living your life in one specific way because of the genitals you were born with. Letting go of the binary will help you to understand your patients who are pansexual. Using a traditional, rigid, and binary lens to try to understand your pansexual patients will only cause you confusion and potentially rupture a therapeutic relationship.

## Defining Pansexuality

As mentioned at the beginning of the chapter, the most common definition for pansexuality is "individuals who feel they are sexually, emotionally, and spiritually capable of being attracted to any person regardless of gender or sex" (Belous and Bauman 2017, p. 58). Pansexual people are open to relationships and sex with people they feel connected to. Connection and attraction are not determined primarily by a potential partner's gender or sex. Each pansexual person determines what they need in order to feel connected to someone. The open nature of the word pansexual allows each individual person to define their sexuality on their own terms.

Some people may gravitate toward this identity because they believe it rejects the idea that gender and genitals are important parts of attraction. Others may claim this identity because they find it inclusive of all genders and not just men and women. Many people who identify as pansexual do so because labeling their sexuality does not feel comfortable, authentic, or valuable. For these people, pansexuality might feel less restrictive than other labels or identities.

Pansexuality can have different meanings for different people, but there are many things that all pansexual people emphasize about what their sexuality means and does not mean. Pansexuality means that an individual is open to the possibility of a romantic or intimate connection with any person. Pansexuality does not mean that an individual *will* have a connection with any person. Pansexuality does not mean that an individual will have a connection with *every* person. A pansexual person can have preferences, different levels of attraction to different people, and, at times, no attraction to certain people. Past or current sexual or romantic behavior does not have any bearing on whether or not a person identifies as pansexual. A person can be a virgin and still identify as pansexual because they are attracted to and open to connections with any person regardless of gender or sex.

The fluidity of sexuality is a very important concept for pansexual people. Sexuality is often viewed as rigid, fixed, and binary. Pansexual people do not believe they have to identify the same way their entire lives or be defined in opposition to or comparison with other identities. In sum, pansexual people are attracted to whomever they are attracted. They do not prioritize gender or sex in relationships, and their sexuality does not have to stay the same their entire lives. They will have sex with the people with whom they want to have sex. This does not mean that they will have sex with everyone or have more sex than most people.

## Realities for Pansexual People

As health care providers, we often rely on research, data, and evidence-based practices to inform our work and to make sure we are providing the best care for the populations we serve. This may lead some providers to wonder: If pansexuality has a different meaning for each person, how do we understand the needs of the pansexual population? How do we generalize our work to a population of people who defy generalization?

There is some information about who is more likely to identify as pansexual and specific challenges pansexual people face. It is important to keep in mind, however, that there is no universal experience for pansexual people. Different pansexual people will have different stories, needs and challenges.

Pansexuality has become increasingly popular with younger members of the community. "Scholars speculate pansexuality is gaining acceptance and membership—especially among millennials and 'generation Z'—due to the broad and flexible definition allowing for the freedom of choice and self-identification regarding sexual expression" (Belous and Bauman 2017, p. 60). Generation Z refers to individuals who are younger than the millennial generation (generally, individuals born in the late 1990s onward). Pansexuality has become more visible after a number of celebrities, such as Janelle Monáe, Miley Cyrus, and Jazz Jennings, came out as pansexual (Belous and Bauman 2017; Bonos 2018). These celebrities emphasize their willingness to find love and connection with any person who is willing to love and connect with them. They also challenge the need and pressure to label one's sexuality.

People who identify as pansexual often find community and support on the Internet. Blogs and online forums such as Tumblr, LiveJournal, Reddit, and WordPress can be extremely valuable resources for people who identify as pansexual. It is not uncommon for people to come out as pansexual in online communities before coming out to friends and family members in person. Online communities may even feel safer than LGBTQ community and health centers. This is due to stigma and lack of understanding that can occur within the LGBTQ community.

There are many misconceptions about pansexuality among people who are attracted to only one gender or sex (heterosexual, gay, and lesbian people). A pansexual person may be seen as going through a phase, as being confused or promiscuous, or coasting on straight privilege (if they are in a seemingly straight relationship). Pansexual people may face hostility from heterosexual people because of homophobia and perceived promiscuity. They may face hostility from gay- and lesbian-identified individuals who are protective of queer spaces and view pansexual people as confused about their sexuality. These misconceptions about pansexuality may cause pansexual people to avoid LGBTQ centers and health care providers. Additionally, a pansexual person may not come out to their providers for fear of being judged or misunderstood.

If a man identifies as heterosexual, this means he is attracted to and open to having sex and relationships with women. If he gets married to a woman, he can still be attracted to women other than his wife. This does not go away when he gets married. These feelings do not make him more likely to cheat; he has made a choice to be monogamous. He can still be attracted to other women and also stay faithful to his wife. If a man identifies as pansexual, this means he is attracted to and open to having sex and relationships with people regardless of gender. If he gets married to a woman, he can still be attracted to other people of any gender. This also does not make him more likely to cheat because, again, he has made a choice to be monogamous. He can still be attracted to people regardless of gender and stay faithful to his wife.

## Questions Well-Meaning People Ask

**What is the difference between pansexuality and bisexuality?**

*Pansexuality* and *bisexuality* are both labels for people who are attracted to more than one gender or sex. Binary thought has taught us to understand sexuality in rigid and concrete terms. Just as we have been taught to understand such categories as gay or straight and man or woman, we want to try to understand people as being either bisexual or pansexual. However, the truth is that when asked "bisexual or pansexual?" many people answer "bisexual *and* pansexual" or "sometimes bisexual, sometimes pansexual." Some pansexual people will identify as bisexual or queer depending on whom they are speaking with or what type of situation they are in. If a pansexual person believes that the person they are speaking with is not familiar with the term pansexuality, they may identify as bisexual. This is because bisexuality is a more commonly known identity.

Historically, bisexuality has been defined as an attraction to both men and women. However, as people began to understand that there are more than two genders, the definition of bisexuality shifted to be more inclusive of people who exist outside of the gender binary. The binary definition of bisexuality is individuals who are attracted to both men and women. In nonbinary terms, bisexuality means an attraction to more than one gender or sex. This is a small but crucial difference. The binary definition acknowledges only two genders. The nonbinary definition includes multiple genders and sexes. It includes people who identify as transgender, bigender, agender, genderqueer, and genderfluid, to name a few. Many people who identify as bisexual are attracted to people of various genders, not solely people within the gender binary.

In an effort to explain the difference between pansexuality and bisexuality, people often fall back on the binary definition of bisexuality. It is common to find articles that say bisexuality means an attraction to just men and women, whereas pansexuality includes an attraction to all genders and sexes. This is incorrect. Both identities are inclusive of all genders.

The definitions of both identities are similar, but there are definitely differences among those who identify as pansexual and those who identify as bisexual. Some research suggests that pansexual-identified people tend to be younger than people who identify as bisexual (Morandini et al. 2016). Some research suggests people who identify as bisexual may be "more likely than individuals identifying as pansexual to state a preference for one group over another, and to indicate a preferred identity for their partner" (Galupo et al. 2016, p. 119). Additionally, because pansexuality is a lesser-known identity, pansexual people typically experience more stigma than those who identify as bisexual. This may be due to the fact that although the binary definition of bisexuality is inaccurate, it still has a binary definition. Therefore, people who see the world through a binary lens tend to be more accepting of bisexual people than of pansexual people.

Although bisexuality is an identity in and of itself, it is also used as an umbrella term for all people who are attracted to more than one gender. Researchers refer to pansexuality as part of the *bisexual umbrella* (Flanders et al. 2017; Galupo et al. 2016). In research, pansexuality and bisexuality are often grouped together, and most attempts to understand pansexual people will include information from bisexual individuals as well. It is not uncommon for pansexual people to be regarded as part of the bi+ community, a grouping of individuals who are attracted to more than one gender or sex. This community can include people who identify as pansexual, bisexual, queer, omnisexual, or any other identity that involves relationships with more than one gender or sex. The grouping of these identities has both benefits and drawbacks. Being grouped together with bisexual people can provide community, help people find commonalities, and assist with advocacy and activism. However, it can also lead to the erasure of the specific needs and stories of pansexual people.

Each person who identifies as pansexual will have a personal and individual reason for why this label resonates with them. If you are interested in why the person you are working with has claimed the identity of pansexual as opposed to bisexual, it may be valuable to respectfully ask.

**If pansexual people are open to a connection with anyone, does this include children?**

No. Pansexual people are open to an emotional, physical, and/or spiritual connection with any consenting adult regardless of gender or sex. This does not include children, inanimate objects, animals, or dead bodies.

**Do pansexual people have more sex or riskier sex than people who are attracted to only one gender?**

Pansexual people are not necessarily more sexually active than people who are attracted to one gender. Pansexuality does not imply promiscuity or risky sexual behavior. In fact, a person does not have to be sexually active at all in order to identify as pansexual. A person can identify as pansexual if they are merely willing and open to attraction an+d connections with people of all sexes and genders.

**Are all pansexual people non-monogamous?**

Monogamy is one way of having a romantic relationship. When two people are monogamous, they romantically love only each other and have sex only with each other. Non-monogamy describes relationships that do not adhere to this standard. A pansexual person may be open to non-monogamous or polyamorous relationships. Pansexuality, however, does not automatically imply non-monogamy. There are many people who identify as pansexual who are engaged in or interested in monogamous relationships.

**Are pansexual people attracted to everyone?**

Just as a lesbian will not be attracted to every woman she meets or a heterosexual woman will not be attracted to every man she meets, a pansexual person will not be attracted to every person that they meet. A pansexual person can have preferences, different levels of attraction to people of different genders or sexes, and no attraction to certain people.

**Does the gender of a person's partner change or impact their pansexual identity?**

A person's sexual identity does not change when they enter into a relationship. A man can be in a relationship with another man and still identify as pansexual. A person's identity can be fluid and changing over time, but their identity depends on them. It does not depend on who they are in a relationship with.

**If pansexual people are attracted to people regardless of sex or gender, do they still recognize the importance that sex or gender identity may have to other people?**

Pansexual people do not prioritize sex or gender when making decisions about who they are attracted to or who they have sex with. However, pansexual people do acknowledge the importance of gender in everyday life. They understand that gender identity and expression are important ways in which people express themselves.

**Do you have to have a certain gender identity to be pansexual?**

No. Pansexual people can have any gender identity, and there is no specific gender identity required in order to identify as pansexual. Pansexual people can be transgender, cisgender, nonbinary, genderfluid, agender, and so on.

# Themes That May Emerge in Therapy

## COUNTERTRANSFERENCE

There are countless reasons why a pansexual person might seek out therapy. They may want support coming out to their friends and family. They may want support communicating with partners of different sexual orientations or tools for coping with depression and anxiety due to stigma. They may want to talk about challenges related to their sexuality, or they may not. There is no way of telling if someone is pansexual by looking at them, so sexuality is something that should be asked about and incorporated into every initial meeting with a new patient.

Patients may also be curious about their therapist's sexual identity and will most likely be looking for hints or signs that indicate whether or not you will be affirming (Baldwin et al. 2017). Each clinician has their own boundaries regarding disclosure. It is by no means mandatory to disclose your own sexuality or background to a patient. However, your patients are already making judgments about you and wondering whether or not you will understand them. Why not speak openly about your sexuality? It may be valuable to challenge yourself to have an open discussion with patients about your own identities and what you bring into the therapy room. More often than not, discussions about a clinician's identities are met with gratitude from patients. Of course, these conversations must be approached in an ethical, thoughtful, and appropriate way.

It is crucial to pay attention to the thoughts and feelings that come up for you when sitting with any patient in therapy. It is important to have some information about yourself to offer and to be aware of what you feel comfortable with when interacting with different patients. Are you someone who likes definitive answers and universal truths? Do you feel uncomfortable with ambiguity? Is it important for you to have all the answers and information that your patients may need? These traits are not bad traits to have, and they most likely make you a great health care provider. It is important to seek out information that will help your patients. However, these traits may also make it difficult for you to sit with a pansexual patient because they may lead to feelings of frustration or embarrassment about not having all of the answers for the person.

If you are unsure about what thoughts and feelings may come up for you when meeting with a pansexual person, then ask yourself what comes up for you when reading this chapter. There may be some feelings of annoyance about the terms used or about the lack of concrete definitions. You may still be wondering about what the *actual* difference is between pansexuality and bisexuality. You may feel uncomfortable about having to ask each pansexual patient what pansexuality means for them. All of these feelings provide great information about yourself and how you work. What do you do when these feelings of discomfort and frustration arise in you? Do you continue to ask questions until you get an answer that makes you feel better? Do you feel the urge to argue? Do you feel shut down? Are you able to sit with discomfort and embrace gray areas? Could you adopt a respectful curiosity about your patient's experience in the world? Would it be acceptable to you to ask your patient to help you understand them better?

Perhaps these feelings of frustration are coming up because of your own upbringing. How were you taught about sex? How were you treated with regard to your sexual orientation or gender identity? What messages did you receive about sexuality growing up? Your own sexual history is most definitely present in the room as you meet with your patients.

You may feel compelled to stop talking or asking questions for fear you will offend your patient. However, asking questions about what a patient's identity means to them can lead to fruitful and positive therapeutic conversations. It is extremely important to approach diverse sexualities from a place of curiosity and validation. A patient will feel hopeful and motivated if they feel their provider is making an effort to understand them. Additionally, asking your patient about their pansexual identity supports the idea that not all pansexual people are the same and that you cannot understand a person on the basis of a label. Being asked about their sexuality in a genuine and open way is an important factor in a patient's decision to come out to their provider (Baldwin et al. 2017). If a patient is not asked about their sexuality in a genuine way, they may not come out at all.

Tuning in to how you feel when reading this chapter can also be important for understanding what pansexual people face in the world. If you find yourself wishing this identity could be easier to understand or wishing your patient would just pick one gender to be attracted to, other people in their life have probably already expressed this to them. Reactions like these can make pansexual people feel that they are too much or too difficult to understand. It may be helpful to ask your patient if they have had to deal with such feelings from family members, friends, or people in the LGBTQ+ community.

Although countertransference is a vital part of therapy with any patient, it is particularly important to keep in mind when working with a demographic or population that is new to you. Asking yourself questions about your countertransference will keep your own history, thoughts, and feelings in the forefront of your mind, and these insights will help immensely in building connections with your pansexual patients.

## MINORITY STRESS

Minority stress theory suggests that someone who belongs to an oppressed group will have more stress and therefore more health issues than those who are not in an oppressed group (Borgogna et al. 2019). For example, the stress connected to being gay will put gay people at greater risk than straight people for mental and physical health issues. According to this theory, everyone in the LGBTQ[2]IAP acronym will have more barriers to mental and physical health than do heterosexual cisgender people. Because pansexual people are a minority within the LGBTQ+ community, they will experience greater stress than do lesbian and gay people. According to this theory, pansexual people are a minority within a minority.

In a study comparing the mental health of people with various sexual identities, pansexual participants reported more depression and anxiety than did gay and lesbian participants (Borgogna et al. 2019). This will most definitely come up in your work with pansexual people. The stress of being in a stigmatized group leads to increased mental health challenges. It can also lead to the avoidance of health care for fear of being misunderstood or judged by health care providers. If a pansexual person seeks out health care, they are less likely than other members of the community to disclose their sexual identity (Baldwin et al. 2017).

Pansexual people often face rejection from other members of the LGBTQ+ community. Even within the community, there is fear of people who are attracted to more than one gender. There are judgments about pansexual people being promiscuous, more likely to carry STDs, or confused about what their "real" sexual orientation is. Feeling isolated by the community they are supposed to be a part of can lead to depression in pansexual people. When working with a pansexual person, it will be helpful to assist them in finding a community where they feel accepted. Keep in mind that online communities can be very supportive and informative.

If you are aware of the concerns that pansexual people have about health care providers, you can include some things in your interactions with patients that may help them feel more comfortable. In order to combat the stigma that pansexual people face, you can show them that you are non-judgmental and do not assume anything about them on the basis of their sexuality. Assure your patient that you are aware that being pansexual does mean someone is promiscuous or more prone to STDs. Keep in mind that not all pansexual people will come out to you at your first meeting, so consider making the following actions part of your practice with all patients, regardless of their identity:

- If your patient is talking about a partner, ask for the partner's pronouns or use gender-neutral language when referring to their partner. This will indicate to a patient that you are not assuming their sexuality.
- Ask about the patient's sexuality. Ask about how they define their identity and what their identity means to them.
- Ask about the places where the patient feels safe and supported. Ask them what helps them feel safe and supported.
- Provide appropriate sexual health information. For example, do not automatically suggest birth control to a sexually active woman. She may not be having the kind of sex that puts her at risk of getting pregnant. She may not have the body parts necessary to become pregnant.
- Continuously check in about sexuality. This will show your patients that you understand that sexuality can be fluid and can change over time.
- Although people are definitely the experts on their own experiences and stories, they may not be informed about everything. You might need to provide your patients with psychoeducation about the fluidity of gender and sexuality. It may be a huge relief to a patient to learn that they do not have to identify the same way their whole life.

If pansexual people experience more stress due to their minority status within the LGBTQ+ community, actions like the ones above can help relieve that stress by helping your patients feel understood and accepted. Opening up conversations about sexuality can foster a sense of safety and help a patient feel less like an outsider. By contrast, avoiding these conversations can increase feelings of minority stress by sending the message that you don't care about your patient's identity because it is not well known.

## RELATIONSHIPS AND INVISIBILITY

If a man identifies as heterosexual and is married to a woman, he can still be attracted to women other than his wife. If a man identifies as pansexual and is married to a woman, he can still be attracted to other people regardless of gender. On meeting both of these men and their wives, you might assume that both men are heterosexual. We often make assumptions about people's sexual identity on the basis of their partners. However, one of these men does not identify as heterosexual. He may have had relationships with people who do not identify as women. He may be very proud of this identity and should not have to give it up because of his choice of partner. Attraction to people does not go away when someone is in a monogamous relationship, and this is true of people who identify as pansexual as well as those who identify as heterosexual.

In therapy, it is important to acknowledge the challenges that arise for pansexual people in relationships. Pansexual people may feel that their identity is invisible if they are consistently being labeled on the basis of whom they are dating. This may be a main reason that pansexual people seek therapy. People identify as pansexual because it is important for them to communicate that their sexuality is fluid and nonbinary. A pansexual person remains pansexual regardless of who their partner is. It can be invalidating and shortsighted to assume someone is gay or straight simply because of who they are in a relationship with.

Pansexuality is often made invisible in history. People who may have been pansexual icons, such as Freddie Mercury or Marlene Dietrich, are often labeled as gay or straight in the media (Niki 2017). These icons are important for pansexual people because they inform others about the identity and show that pansexual people are capable of accomplishing great things. They give pansexual youth people to look to for guidance. Therefore, pansexual representation in the media is crucial for acceptance and protection.

Another challenge that may come up in therapy is a pansexual person's partner having concerns about the pansexual person's sexuality. It is common for a partner to be worried that they cannot provide everything that their pansexual partner may want or need sexually. There may be fears that a pansexual person is more likely to cheat because they are attracted to more than one gender. This can lead to feelings of guilt, shame, and disappointment for the pansexual partner. There are plenty of ways that pansexual people can get their needs met in monogamous relationships, and in order for this to happen, they must be able to communicate with their partner openly and honestly, without being met with suspicion or blame. In therapy, you can help your pansexual patients by validating their identity and assisting them in exploring how they might be able to get their needs met in relationships. You may also offer information about non-monogamy, which can be a liberating and valuable option for couples who have different sexual orientations.

Pansexual people may also face rejection from the LGBTQ+ community. A pansexual person in a relationship with a heterosexual person may feel isolated from the LGBTQ+ community if their relationship is deemed straight. It also may be difficult for pansexual people to navigate and accept the privilege of being seen as straight by society. The privilege pansexual people hold when in a seemingly straight relationship cannot be denied. They are not harassed when they walk down the street, and they can choose whether or not to disclose their identity. It may be helpful to look at your pansexual patients' privileged and subordinated identities and how these identities affect them.

It is important for pansexual people to feel understood and accepted by their communities. Assisting your pansexual patients in finding community will be very helpful in your work. Support your patient in locating or organizing events for the pansexual community. Pansexual Pride Day is on December 8, and Pansexual Day of Visibility is on May 24. These days help spread awareness and acceptance both outside and within the LGBTQ+ community.

## Conclusion

Conversations about relationships are central to therapy. If you are aware of some of the challenges pansexual people may face in relationships, you will be better equipped to help your patients navigate these challenges. Keep in mind that a pansexual person is still pansexual regardless of the sex or gender of the person with whom they decide to have a relationship. Understand that pansexual people may have partners who are attracted to only one gender. Your patient may need support in communicating their needs to their partner and managing guilt or shame that comes up for them in their relationship. Finally, a pansexual person may feel isolated from the LGBTQ+ community, especially if they are in a relationship that is deemed heterosexual. They may need help finding resources or a community that feels accepting and validating.

## FIVE TAKE-HOME POINTS

- Pansexual people are open to relationships and intimacy with any consenting adult they feel a connection with regardless of that person's gender or sex.

- Pansexual people will not be attracted to any person or every person that they meet. They can have preferences and types and can feel no attraction at all to some people.

- The definitions of *pansexuality* and *bisexuality* are very similar. Both identities mean that a person is attracted to more than one gender or sex. At times, people use the two identities interchangeably. Each person will have their own individual reasons why they identify as pansexual rather than bisexual.

- Sexuality is fluid for pansexual people. It can change over time.

- Pansexuality can be hard to understand because people are taught about sexuality in binary terms. If we learn about the complexity and variety of bodies, gender, and sex, it might be easier to understand pansexuality. Using nonbinary language will help you understand your pansexual patients.

## Resources

Pansexuality is often grouped with bisexuality, and pansexual people are regarded as part of the bi+ community. Note that many of the online resources that may be helpful for you and your pansexual patients are geared toward the bi+ community.

Bi+, GLAAD, www.glaad.org/tags/bi-0. This website includes blogs and articles geared toward bi+ people covering topics such as health care, discovering one's pansexual identity, and the invisibility pansexual people feel in relationships.

Bisexual Resource Center, https://biresource.org. This website is a resource for members of the bi+ community to find groups and support in their area. It includes information on the bi+ community and a helpful video about pansexuality and bisexuality.

## References

Baldwin A, Dodge B, Schick V, et al: Health and identity-related interactions between lesbian, bisexual, queer and pansexual women and their healthcare providers. Cult Health Sex 19(11):1181–1196, 2017 28318398

Belous CK, Bauman ML: What's in a name? Exploring pansexuality online. J Bisex 17(1):58–72, 2017

Bonos L: Janelle Monáe comes out as "pansexual." What does that mean? Washington Post, April 26, 2018. Available at: www.washingtonpost.com/news/soloish/wp/2018/04/26/janelle-monae-comes-out-as-pansexual-what-does-that-mean. Accessed January 23, 2019.

Borgogna NC, McDermott RC, Aita SL, et al: Anxiety and depression across gender and sexual minorities: implications for transgender, gender nonconforming, pansexual, demisexual, asexual, queer, and questioning individuals. Psychol Sex Orientat Gend Divers 6(1):54–63, 2019

Flanders CE, LeBreton ME, Robinson M, et al: Defining bisexuality: young bisexual and pansexual people's voices. J Bisex 17(1):39–52, 2017

Galupo MP, Ramirez JL, Pulice-Farrow L: "Regardless of their gender": descriptions of sexual identity among bisexual, pansexual, and queer identified individuals. J Bisex 17(1):108–124, 2016

Morandini JS, Blaszczynski A, Dar-Nimrod I: Who adopts queer and pansexual sexual identities? J Sex Res 54(7):911–922, 2016 27911091

Niki D: Now you see me, now you don't: addressing bisexual invisibility in relationship therapy. Sex Relation Ther 33(1–2):45–57, 2017

# Chapter 10

# Ally

## *The Second A in LGBTQ²IAPA*

ANGELIKI PESIRIDOU, M.D.
SERENA M. CHANG, M.D.

> In the end,
> we will remember not the words of our enemies,
> but the silence of our friends.
>
> *Martin Luther King Jr.*

## Psychological and Cultural Context

The first time I was in contact with the LGBTQ+ community was in medical school. In the early 1990s, when I was in my early 20s, some of my boyfriend's friends were gay men. I remember one of them, who was in his mid-40s, wearing a wedding band (prior to the legalization of gay marriage), pretending to be married and straight in order to feel more comfortable at work. At that time, I was not aware of the depth of the struggles of being a member of a sexual minority group. Twenty years later, most of my closest friends and co-workers are part of the LGBTQ+ community. I now know much more than I did in the 1990s and proudly identify as a straight ally.

The definition of the word *ally*, according to Dictionary.com, is "a person, group, or nation that is associated with another or others for some common cause or purpose." When referring to LGBTQ+ allies, I would add that the term refers to straight privilege with respect to a minority group.

Because we live in a heteronormative society, being born heterosexual and cisgender grants one privileges (Eliason et al. 2013; McGeorge and Stone Carlson 2011). We all carry automatic unconscious beliefs that heterosexuality and cisgender identity are the norm. Institutions, government, the health system, and the educational system promote a heterosexual, cisgender lifestyle with their policies and actions. Heterosexual cisgender people enjoy assumed civil rights, societal benefits, and advantages based solely on their sexual orientation and gender identity (Mathers et al. 2018).

Everyone has been taught that being straight and cisgender is "normal"; therefore, everything else is abnormal or wrong. Even the word *straight* means properly positioned, undeviating, and linear, implying that anything else is crooked or twisted. Few heterosexual cisgender people wonder why they were born heterosexual or are asked to change their sexuality. Straight people do not question their heterosexuality, or their gender identity, or have to defend it. For example, people do not think twice if a heterosexual person wants to express affection with their partner in public. Straight cisgender people are not worried about repercussions if people know their sexual orientation or gender identity. They do not need to hide.

For members of the LGBTQ+ community, these worries are common, and they also must deal with lack of acceptance from mainstream society starting in early childhood. Many of them fall under the category of gender or sexual minorities and include people who identify as gay, lesbian, bisexual, transgender, or questioning their sexuality. Unlike heterosexual children, LGBTQ+ children have to hide their identity either at home or at school or both.

The Centers for Disease Control and Prevention reported that LGBTQ+ students are 30.5% more likely than their heterosexual peers at the same age to feel sad or hopeless, 13.6% more likely to be victims of sexual violence, 23% more likely to attempt suicide, and twice as likely to experiment with hallucinogenic drugs (Landry 2017). Anti-LGBTQ+ remarks often are not addressed in school, and anti-LGBTQ+ jokes and anti-LGBTQ+ name-calling often are not stopped in the classroom setting. Not taking any action in school or at home is still an action, and doing so silently confirms the anti-LGBTQ+ environment and ideas. In addition, there is a great lack of LGBTQ-related themes in curricula. All of these conditions strengthen an LGBTQ+ student's feeling of potential danger and nonacceptance and the need to stay closeted

(Byrd and Hays 2012; Landry 2017; Robinson and Espelage 2011), as shown in the following vignette:

> Nikki is a 7-year-old genderfluid student who was born biologically male and presents as genderfluid at school, sometimes dressing in skirts and dresses. Nikki had consistent and ongoing problems being bullied by other students. One of the biggest problems was Nikki's hesitation about going to the boys' bathroom. The teachers allowed Nikki to go to the teacher's bathroom, which some people might judge as an appropriate accommodation. However, a school that is a real ally to LGBTQ+ students would have gender-neutral bathrooms for everyone. That would be an example of an inclusive school.

As LGBTQ people grow up and enter the work environment, they are still in danger. There is no federal statute addressing employment discrimination based on sexual orientation or gender identity (Brooks and Edwards 2009; Gates 2011). Many people at work are closeted, keeping their personal lives private, afraid to share details about their partners, hobbies, or vacations. Furthermore, many people of trans experience are often misgendered, discriminated against, and bullied. The problems increase if they transition on the job. Many people of trans experience endure the harassment in silence or choose to change jobs and start fresh at a different job that is unaware of their transition. LGBTQ+ people deserve to feel included, safe, and equal to the rest of their coworkers. They deserve family leave when their partners get sick and should be able to bring their partners to work functions without worrying about criticism or discrimination from their coworkers and superiors.

> Maria is a lesbian woman who has health insurance through work. Maria and her partner, Anna, want to have a child. According to the company's rules, health insurance will not cover the process for Maria to get pregnant by donor sperm because they are a same-sex couple. Unlike their heterosexual colleagues, Maria and Anna have to save up money themselves and pay out of pocket in order to be able to have a child as a couple. Furthermore, Anna is not biologically linked to the child, so legally she has no parental rights if Maria and Anna split up.

Furthermore, when it comes to health care, LGBTQ+ people are heavily discriminated against (Eliason et al. 2013;

Kano et al. 2016; Landry 2017). Currently, in many rural and certain urban areas, health care providers lack education about, terminology for, and basic understanding of LGBTQ+ culture. From the very first office visit, LGBTQ+ patients encounter incorrect pronoun use and an environment that does not allow for gender fluidity. Medical staff's thinking in terms of sex assigned at birth and gender as a binary concept already creates discomfort for many LGBTQ+ patients even before they have a chance to address the reason for their visit.

Thinking in heteronormative ways about sexual and social history prevents a thorough health evaluation and screening. LGBTQ+ patients are not offered appropriate screenings, education, and preventive care, such as contraception and pre-exposure prophylaxis for HIV, anal Pap smears, and frequent screenings for sexually transmitted infections (Eliason et al. 2013; Kano et al. 2016; Landry 2017). Because of discrimination, many patients are afraid to disclose their HIV status, and therefore, they avoid necessary medical follow-ups.

> John went home to a rural area in Alabama, where he grew up, to visit his parents. While there, he got sick with an upper respiratory infection. When John went to the clinic in the small town where his parents live, he did not disclose to the doctor that he is HIV positive and the medication that he is taking for HIV—information that is directly relevant to treatment. John not only feared judgment from the doctor and the staff but did not even trust that the information would stay private. This speaks to the trauma and mistrust that LGBTQ+ people experience in the medical system as a whole.

Medical providers often come across as dismissive and judgmental. The "don't ask/don't tell" model has been ineffective. It is the duty of clinics as a whole to create an LGBTQ-friendly environment. LGBTQ+ patients deserve equal treatment, empathy, and the same compassion as everyone else.

For all the above reasons, it is extremely important to be a straight ally. Being a straight ally comes in many forms: some allies actively support the LGBTQ+ community through their work, protest, political beliefs, and everyday lives, but you can also be an ally by paying attention to smaller things, such as the following examples. Every small step matters.

- Use the singular pronoun *they* if you do not know someone's gender

- Use more inclusive words, such as *partner* instead of *husband* or *wife* (for people of all orientations)
- Be open to learning more about the LGBTQ+ community by doing research and asking friends for information
- Be open to input
- Apologize if you accidentally offend a friend or a coworker; don't react defensively if you do offend them
- Address anti-LGBTQ+ jokes or remarks: gently explain why the person's comment is offensive to you and try to engage them in a conversation about why
- Educate coworkers, friends, and children about the LGBTQ+ community; social media is one way to educate and engage people
- Have a sticker of the LGBTQ flag at your workplace

## Questions Well-Meaning People Ask

**I am straight and a cisgender woman. Is it OK for me to speak up about a group I am not part of?**

Historically, many oppressed groups have been supported by allies: think about the civil rights movement. When it comes to oppression and discrimination, all support is welcome and very much needed. Allies are some of the most effective and powerful voices in all movements.

**Where do I start?**

The first step to being an ally is to listen. When you take the time to truly hear others and try to understand them, people notice. All of us feel like an "outsider" at some point in our lives. Being an ally means listening nonjudgmentally with curiosity and empathy. Being an ally means leaving space for people to find their voice. Many LGBTQ+ people do not talk and instead scan the room to get a sense of how they will be received. As a person who is not a sexual and gender minority, you probably have had the space to speak up. By not taking up all the space, we allow space for LGBTQ+ people to feel safe and speak up. Making assumptions and speaking for them actually proves your privilege (Mathers et al. 2018). Being an ally means supporting by listening and not speaking up *for* them.

**If I am vocal about LGBTQ+ rights and "come out" as an ally, will people think I am LGBTQ+?**

That is a possibility. It can be uncomfortable at first, but this is an opportunity to experience firsthand the challenges LGBTQ+ people deal with all the time, which can actually make you a better ally. The trade-off is that it will make LGBTQ+ people feel comfortable and supported, and there are also many more allies out there who will support you. The gain is much greater than the risk.

**How do I become more comfortable talking about LGBTQ+ issues?**

The answer is simple: educate, educate, educate yourself. Start with learning the language, then improve your equality literacy and strive to understand gender and sexual orientation fluidity. The more you learn about LGBTQ+ issues, the more comfortable you will feel when discussing these issues with people both within and outside the LGBTQ+ community.

**What if I say something offensive or misgender someone?**

Do not get defensive. Listen and apologize. Ask questions respectfully and educate yourself.

**How do I address anti-LGBTQ+ comments, jokes, policies, or behaviors without coming across as confrontational?**

Many people do not address anti-LGBTQ behavior because they do not want others to feel uncomfortable or because they fear being excluded. It is appropriate to address the behavior politely and to state facts. Address the behavior, not the person: "I think the joke you just made was homophobic" instead of "You are homophobic." Explain why you are speaking up: "As a straight ally, I think it is very important to speak up." Listen to the other person's argument, whether they apologize or disagree. Thank the person for their time and offer the opportunity to discuss the topic again at another time if the person is interested.

**How do I incorporate being an ally in my everyday life?**

Educate yourself, be open to criticism, and try to be nondefensive. Use inclusive language and incorporate LGBTQ+ symbols, such as the flag, in your workspace or post an article about LGBTQ+ care in your social media feed.

**What does it mean to be an ally?**

An ally wants to learn, address barriers, and address disparity. Here are some tips:

1. Examine your own prejudice
2. Leave space for LGBTQ+ voices
3. Listen and learn the facts
4. Understand the language
5. Stop anti-LGBTQ+ behavior
6. Be public
7. Train and educate others

**How do I make my clinic LGBTQ+ friendly?**

Place stickers and posters in the waiting area indicating that
your clinic is a safe place. Change the electronic medical records system to allow for more inclusive gender options (female, male, other) and more options on name (preferred
name, insurance card name). Provide gender-neutral bath-
rooms. Offer frequent staff trainings, and change Human Resources rules if they are not LGBTQ+ friendly.

**How do I make a school environment more inclusive?**

Place stickers and posters in the office. Provide straight-gay
alliance clubs (Poteat et al. 2013) and gender-neutral bath-
rooms. Establish LGBTQ+ curricula in classes such as health,
biology, and history/social studies and ensure school counselor competency (Byrd and Hays 2012).

# Themes that May Emerge in Therapy

Now that you have read this book, you are armed with the resources needed to fill in any gaps in basic knowledge in your
work with LGBTQ-identified patients. All that remains is to
create the human connection. For cisgender, heterosexual-
identified providers, one of the biggest challenges is striking
the right balance in their approach and addressing issues of
transference and countertransference. Just as a therapist
quickly recognizes that there is no one-size-fits-all approach
to patients, conversely there is no need to upend one's entire
approach in working with LGBTQ+ individuals. An em-
pathic, open-minded provider already has the tools in their
toolbox to do this work. To varying degrees, all patients come

from a different background from that of the health care provider, and working with someone with a different sexuality or gender identity is comparable to working with a patient of a different race, class, religion, or overall life experience.

That being said, much like engaging in trauma-informed care or being aware of different cultural norms and integrating them into your practice, being an informed practitioner is key. In a similar vein, a common sentiment expressed by white Americans is that they grew up in households in which race and its impact on individuals, culture, and society, were not discussed. Because white is the majority racial group, many Americans grow up thinking that white is "normal," the default racial makeup. Until relatively recently, mainstream media worked from this assumption, which was reflected in many aspects of culture: greeting cards, magazines, children's books, movies. When confronted with the reality that a large portion of the population was not represented in this vision, the reaction of many in the majority gave rise to the notion of "color-blindness," that everyone should be treated the same regardless of their skin color. However, this approach fails in its lack of nuance and awareness, namely, in its failure to recognize privilege, the idea that not everyone begins life with the same advantages. What is needed is not equality, in which everyone is treated identically, but equity, which seeks to offset privilege (Figure 10–1).

For people who identify as part of the majority group of heterosexuality, the idea that everyone else is like them is called *heteronormativity*. Thus, for allies, the process of greater understanding begins with 1) awareness of how their own identity as a heterosexual individual has shaped their worldview, 2) understanding of how various institutional systems have enforced heterosexuality as the "norm," and 3) awareness of how this identity has offered various privileges in society. Keep in mind that these topics may seem simple, but heterosexual individuals often find that they have never needed to slow down to consider these ideas—concepts that LGBTQ+ individuals find take up a majority of their daily mind space.

The process of self-awareness begins with considering your worldviews and their origins. Questions to consider include the following:

• Growing up, what did your family teach you about gender and sexuality (e.g., girl vs. boy toys, clothing, dating and marriage, "boys will be boys")?

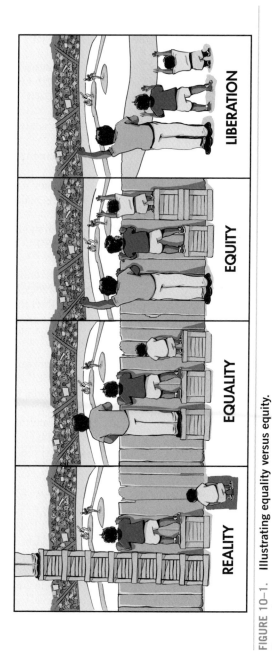

FIGURE 10–1. Illustrating equality versus equity.

*Source.* Interaction Institute for Social Changes. Artist: Angus Maguire. Available at: http://interactioninstitute.org/illustrating-equality-vs-equity.

- What did your religion or spirituality teach you about gender and sexuality?
- What did you learn about gender and sexuality from TV and movies?
- How did you come to view your own gender and sexuality (e.g., when did you "know" you were straight?)?
- What are your thoughts on children raised by LGBTQ+ individuals?
- How would you react if your child came out to you as LGBTQ+?
- When people meet you, how often do they assume the gender of your partner or spouse?
- When you meet someone, how do you know if they are male or female? Do you assume that if someone is male, they have a wife, and vice versa?
- How would you react if you saw a man and a woman showing affection in public versus two men or two women?

Taken on a broader scale, it is easy to see how heteronormativity can lead to institutionalized heterosexism, or the expansion of these ideas on a systemic level greater than the individual level. One only needs to look at recent current events for an idea of what this looks like:

- High-school administrators telling a student that they cannot take their same-sex partner to the prom
- Parents disowning their adolescent child and banning them from the home for being LGBTQ+
- A county clerk refusing to grant marriage certificates for same-sex couples
- A woman being told that she cannot be present with her wife for the birth of their child because she isn't the "real" mother
- Governments openly imprisoning or killing citizens because of their sexual orientation or gender identity

Thus, the role of the clinical care provider is to *not* enact additional trauma onto an already traumatized population by becoming another pillar of institutionalized heterosexism. Sounds challenging? For the individual ally, a simple way to begin is by examining how being a part of the cisgender/heterosexual majority has been an advantage—in other words, admitting one's heterosexual privilege.

When working as an ally with a patient, it's OK to make mistakes. If you do make a mistake, apologize briefly and move on—there is no need to be overly effusive. Setting boundaries and limits is still appropriate—don't patronize or be overly accommodating. When in doubt, ask—your patient, a colleague, another ally, or a member of the LGBTQ+ community. We're all in this together. No one is perfect, and it's always better to clarify than to work from the perspective of a misguided assumption.

## Conclusion

The LGBTQ community is a gender/sexual orientation minority. As such, the members of the community experience prejudice, discrimination, and disadvantage as compared with cisgender, heterosexual people. An ally is a privileged cisgender, heterosexual person who understands this disparity and supports, advocates for, and speaks up for the group. Allies working with the LGBTQ+ community acknowledge heterosexual privilege and address social disparities. Celebrating the diversity of sexual orientation and gender identity creates a safe environment for patients to openly share their struggles and triumphs.

## FIVE TAKE-HOME POINTS

- Being a heterosexual, cisgender person grants you privilege.

- As an ally, recognize that the LGBTQ+ community is a gender/sexual orientation minority.

- Being an ally means educating yourself about the LGBTQ+ community.

- Being an ally means being vocal when needed.

- Being an ally also means leaving space for LGBTQ+ people to speak up.

# Resources

PFLAG (formerly Parents and Friends of Lesbians and Gays), www.pflag.org

GLSEN (formerly Gay, Lesbian and Straight Education Network), www.glsen.org

Atticus Circle, www.atticuscircle.org

World Professional Association for Transgender Health, www.wpath.org

# References

Brooks AK, Edwards K: Allies in the workplace: including LGBT in HRD. Adv Dev Hum Resour 11(1):136–149, 2009

Byrd RJ, Hays D: School counselor competency and lesbian, gay, bisexual, transgender, and questioning (LGBTQ) youth. J School Couns 10(3):1–28, 2012

Eliason MJ, Chinn P, Dibble SL, et al: Open the door for LGBTQ patients. Nursing 43(8):44–50, 2013

Gates TG: Why employment discrimination matters: well-being and the queer employee. J Workplace Rights 16(1):107–128, 2011

Kano M, Silva-Bañuelos AR, Sturm R, et al: Stakeholders' recommendations to improve patient-centered "LGBTQ" primary care in rural and multicultural practices. J Am Board Fam Med 29(1):156–160, 2016 26769889

Landry J: Delivering culturally sensitive care to LGBTQI patients. J Nurse Pract 13(5):342–347, 2017

Mathers LAB, Sumerau JE, Ueno K: "This isn't just another gay group": privileging heterosexuality in a mixed-sexuality LGBTQ advocacy group. J Contemp Ethnogr 47(6):834–864, 2018

McGeorge C, Stone Carlson T: Deconstructing heterosexism: becoming an LGB affirmative heterosexual couple and family therapist. J Marital Fam Ther 37(1):14–26, 2011 21198685

Poteat VP, Sinclair KO, DiGiovanni CD, et al: Gay-straight alliances are associated with student health: a multischool comparison of LGBTQ and heterosexual youth. J Res Adolesc 23(2):319–330, 2013

Robinson JP, Espelage DL: Inequities in educational and psychological outcomes between LGBTQ and straight students in middle and high school. Educ Res 40(7):315–330, 2011

# Index

Page numbers printed in **boldface** type refer to tables and figures.